A View Fr

Dr. August

Keith Publications, LLC
www.keithpublications.com
©2015

Arizona
USA

A View From The Inside

Copyright© 2015

By Dr. Augustine L. Perrotta

Edited by Ray Dyson
Raydyson7@yahoo.com

Cover art by Elisa Elaine Luevanos
www.ladymaverick81.com

Cover art Keith Publications, LLC © 2015
www.keithpublications.com

ISBN: 978-1-62882-093-5

If you are interested in purchasing more works of this nature, please stop by
www.keithpublications.com

Contact information: info@keithpublications.com
Visit us at: www.keithpublications.com

Printed in The United States of America

Dedication

This book is dedicated to my family, especially my wife, Dorothy. During my 32 years of practice, she tolerated my long working hours and almost single-handedly raised our three children, Augie, Grace and Mike. I know I can never make up for all I missed in their lives but, in my retirement, I am trying.

Acknowledgements

I wish to acknowledge the professional editing skills of A.J. Smuskiewicz, the creative artist who illustrated the first 14 chapters. Not only did he grasp the spirit and intent of each vignette, but he created illustrations that captured the essence of the main characters. The artistic talent of Zachary Meyer, who illustrated the front cover and the 15th chapter on a timely schedule, is deeply appreciated. He understood their connotation.

The stimulus to write about the osteopathic medical profession came from Katherine Rollinger, DO, who claimed she always enjoyed my stories about the profession and its history. I am indebted to my brother and roommate for 25 years, Richard C. Perrotta, DO, who convinced me I could be a writer and public speaker since we were boys and never hesitated to be my bedrock of reality. After hearing a verbal account of the content of several chapters of this book, the apt title was suggested by advertising executive Alex Steiner.

That this book has come to print is the result of the guidance and diligence of my agent, Diane S. Nine, Esq., and the editing skills of Ray Dyson, editor for Keith Publications.

Table of Contents

Preface vi

Babe Ruth's Cancer 1

There had to be a Better Way 12

Detroit Never Forgave Him 20

The Deadly Dentist 25

He Could Not Read a Note 39

Snakebite! 44

The Leper on the Bus 53

Bow Ties 58

The Interview 69

Wombmates—Myths and Realities 80

Separate but Equal 113

Humor as Medicine 123

The Father of Bone Marrow Transplantation 154

Jehovah's Witnesses 187

The Oldest Man in the World 224

Preface

In this collection of medically oriented short stories, I have attempted to describe characters and events derived from personal experiences in my life and my connection to them—as I recall them. Certain people, scenes and happenings were selected in an attempt to set the record straight about misinformation, myths, urban legends and junk science surrounding the topics. Several of the chapters reflect the axioms taught to me in early childhood by my mother and father, respectively—"Charity begins at home" and "Do unto others what you would have them do unto you."

It is my intent that you find these anecdotes both entertaining and instructive. To that end, I have tried to fill the stories with trivia relevant and pertinent to the subject matter, while providing a glimpse of human nature and the human condition in a real-world context. My underlying premise is that little happens by chance. I truly believe that coincidence is God's way of staying anonymous.

The title of this book, *A View from the Inside*, was purposefully chosen as a double entendré. It was meant to convey my training and background in internal medicine. I practiced hematology and medical oncology, subspecialties of internal medicine. The origin of internal medicine implies one who diagnoses and treats ailments of the internal organs. There is also the inference that I have insider information about the public and private figures depicted. I have carefully and assiduously attempted to avoid violating patient confidences and the Health Insurance Portability and Accountability Act (HIPAA) regulations. In portraying what I hope is a unique perspective about these encounters and my connection to them; I hope they will be of interest to the reader. Each chapter is a true story and not "based on a true story" as is often claimed about a Hollywood film or television series. The insights and perspectives contained in my stories may be ageless, but the medical facts are not. Although accurate, the medical information should be viewed in the context of the years 1958 to 2014, with updates where pertinent to the story.

I wrote this book as a tribute to the osteopathic medical profession which has given me well beyond the fulfillment of my boyhood dreams and the opportunity to be "a man for others" in the Jesuit tradition. It is also meant to be a legacy to my family, especially my 7 1/2-year-old twin grandsons, Michael and William, and their sister, Caroline Grace, born on January 30, 2013. Perhaps, when they grow up, they will consider becoming osteopathic physicians like their grandfather and granduncle.

It is my wish that this collection of personal experiences be enjoyed by champions of life, religious and civil libertarians, healthcare advocates, sports fans and those who can identify with the topics.

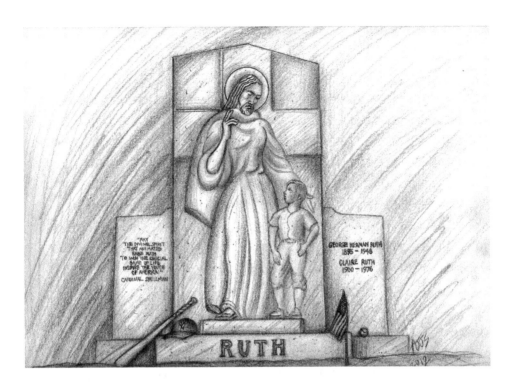

Babe Ruth's Cancer

According to ancient Norse mythology, Valhalla—meaning hall of the slain—is the great hall in the castle of Odin, the chief god of war and death. The souls of warriors who die as heroes in battle dwell eternally in this hall. The valiant warriors are chosen and escorted into the hall by the Valkyries, beautiful young women mounted on winged horses, clad in armor and carrying spears. As they ride forth, their armor causes the strange flickering lights we see as the aurora borealis, or northern lights.

Within the township of Mount Pleasant in Westchester County, New York, lie the rolling hills of an unincorporated hamlet named Valhalla. The name for this hamlet was inspired by the Ring of the Nibelung, a cycle of four operas based on the Norse myth and written by the German composer Richard Wagner between 1869 and 1876. These operas are Das Rheingold (the Rhine Gold), Die Walkure (the Valkyrie), Siegfried, and Die Gotterdammerung (the Twilight of the Gods).

1

The locals use the heroic, mythological name Valhalla to refer to four contiguous cemeteries in Mount Pleasant—Gate of Heaven, Kensico, Mount Pleasant and Mount Eden. Gate of Heaven, about 25 miles north of New York City, is the most scenic and majestic of these cemeteries and falls under the auspices of the Archdiocese of New York. My father, Augustine Vincent, my mother, Louise Ann, and my sister, Carole Ann, are buried there beneath an exquisitely carved gravestone that depicts the Good Samaritan ministering to the robbery victim, with the inscription, "Do unto others as you would have them do unto you." It is an adage that was reinforced many times by my father in my youth. Our family plot accommodates six caskets. I expect to be interred there, as does my brother, Richard Carl.

Many celebrities are reposed in the mausoleums, crypts and graves of Gate of Heaven. But without a map, it is almost impossible to find them among the almost 150,000 gravesites. A few of the famous people interred at Gate of Heaven:

• Fred Allen, comedian
• James Cagney, actor
• James Farley, postmaster general and advisor to President Franklin Roosevelt
• Dorothy Kilgallen, newspaper columnist/television personality
• Wellington Mara, owner of the New York Giants football team
• Billy Martin, baseball player and manager
• Sal Mineo, actor
• Conde Nast, publisher
• Joanne Ortiz-Patino socialite/jetsetter
• Westbrook Pegler, Pulitzer-Prize winning journalist
• Mike Quill, founder of the Transport Workers Union of America
• Dutch Schultz, mobster
• Jimmy Walker, New York City mayor

My mother passed away in 1995 a few days after the 30th anniversary of my sister's death. Our family requested the services of our long-time friend, funeral director William J. Oldani, Jr. He made all the funeral arrangements and offered to drive the hearse containing my mother's coffin for the 900-mile round trip to and from her final resting place at Gate of Heaven. Despite his solitary 11-hour overnight drive, Bill appeared refreshed and impeccably dressed in his classic undertaker's black suit during the funeral Mass in the cemetery's chapel.

Bill was an avid sport's fan, but his true passion was baseball. Besides being a funeral director, he had also been a high school athletics official for more than 30 years, including serving as an umpire for high school baseball. His two sons, William and Matthew, had played both Little League and high school baseball. Bill tried to attend every Detroit Tigers' opening day game, as well as several other Tigers' games each year, and he watched every baseball playoff and World Series game on television. He even traveled to games in neighboring states to watch the Tigers play.

Following my mother's burial service, I thanked Bill profusely for his compassionate and efficient personal services for my family. Knowing his love of baseball, I then asked him if he would like to see Babe Ruth's gravesite. His eyes, still slightly bloodshot from the long overnight drive, suddenly lit up and he excitedly asked, "Is he buried here?"

"Yes," I replied, "Right up the hill. We can walk to it."

As we passed the well-manicured shrubs protecting the gravesite of the Bambino from the road, Bill suddenly exclaimed, "I don't have my camera!"

"Not to worry," I said, "I'll give you my photo collection of the site when we get back home."

As he looked down at the gravesite, he asserted, "I am at the gate of Heaven!"

The gravesite of one of the most revered and recognizable figures in baseball history is suitably memorable. The unusually large granite gravestone is an inspirational work of art. Carved into the vertical stone is a haloed, life-sized figure of Jesus Christ gazing downward at a representation of a child baseball player wearing knickers. The left arm of Christ rests on the youth's shoulder. The face of the stone to the lower left is inscribed with "George Herman Ruth 1895-1948" and "Claire Ruth 1900-1976" (Babe's second wife). On the lower right face of the stone is a quote by Francis Cardinal Spellman, then archbishop of the Diocese of New York (and a fellow alumnus of Fordham College): "May the divine spirit that animated Babe Ruth to win the crucial game of life inspire the youth of America." In the center of the 10-foot-long base of the huge gravestone, in large Roman letters, is the name "RUTH."

On the day we visited the gravesite, a number of items left by other visitors were situated on the ledge of the stone's base. Among these items were a New York Yankees' baseball cap, a youth-sized baseball glove, a baseball, various medals, petition letters for a successful Little League game, and a small American flag.

While growing up in the Bronx, I attended several baseball games at Yankee Stadium ("the House that Ruth Built") with friends. My father took me to only one of those games, when I was 9½ years old. (I have observed that children and the elderly tend to count their birthdays in either whole or half years). It was the most memorable baseball game I ever attended, held on Babe Ruth Day, April 27, 1947. After several baseball executives and former players presented their testimonials, Ruth, a shadow of his former self, was invited to address the crowd at the microphone on home plate. He wore a topcoat to hide how thin and frail he was.

His weak voice was raspy as he said to the crowd:
"Thank you very much, ladies and gentlemen. You know how bad my voice sounds. Well, it feels just as bad. You know this baseball game of ours comes up from the youth. That means the boys. And

4

after you're a boy and grow up to know how to play ball, then you come to the boys you see representing themselves today in your national pastime—the only real game I think in the world, baseball. As a rule, some people think if you give them a football or a baseball or something like that, naturally they're athletes right away, but you can't do that in baseball. You've got to start way down from the bottom when you're six or seven years of age. You can't wait until you're fifteen or sixteen. You gotta let it grow up with you and if you're successful and you try hard enough, you're bound to come out on top just like these boys that come to the top now. There have been so many lovely things said about me and I'm glad that I've had the opportunity to thank everybody. Thank you."

The Sultan of Swat then thanked the previous speakers for their words of praise. And with a wave to the fans, he walked from home plate back to the dugout. He died 16 months later at the age of 53.

The first symptoms of the cancer that took Babe Ruth's life began in the late summer of 1946. His voice became progressively hoarse, and he experienced severe pain behind his left eye. He wrote in his autobiography (The Babe Ruth Story, published in 1948) that his "voice sounded like somebody gargling ashes." The left side of his face swelled so much that his left eye completely closed. His jaw hurt and he had difficulty swallowing, which contributed to his progressive weight loss.

In November 1946, X-ray images revealed a mass at the base of his skull. The mass encompassed three holes in the skull—the jugular foramen, foramen ovale and foramen rotundum—through which emerge the cranial nerves. Ruth was treated with external beam radiotherapy, in which X rays are directed at tumors in the body to kill the cancer cells. The treatment initially resulted in some relief of Ruth's pain and swelling. In December, however, a mass appeared on the left side of his neck. An attempt at surgical removal of the bulk of the mass was unsuccessful, because the tumor was wrapped around the external carotid artery. The surgeons had to tie off the artery, because encroachment by the tumor put it at risk for rupture and exsanguination (extensive loss of blood) from a blowout. The cancer also invaded the lymph nodes on the left side of his neck.

In June 1947, Ruth received another course of radiation treatment, as well as a female hormone, in an attempt to control the growth of the tumor. This treatment was followed by use of an experimental chemotherapy drug that had shown some success in mice. The drug, called teropterin, was the first in a class of antitumor chemotherapy agents known as folic acid antagonists. The agents work by blocking the ability of cancer cells to use folic acid (a B-complex vitamin) in their metabolism. A subsequent derivative—that is, an analogue—of teropterin is methotrexate, which is used today not only as an antitumor and antileukemia drug, but also as an immune system suppressant for patients with benign autoimmune diseases.

Ruth responded dramatically to the experimental drug. The mass in his neck disappeared. Not only did he gain weight, but he also experienced substantial reductions in his hoarseness and face pain. Sadly, these gains were short-lived, and his symptoms soon returned. By June 1948, he had received more irradiation, and radioactive gold seeds had been implanted in his neck.

Because hoarseness heralded the onset of Ruth's disease and plagued him throughout his illness, his doctors assumed he had cancer of the larynx (voicebox). This diagnosis was reinforced when Ruth admitted to using tobacco and drinking alcohol since he was a child. He once told a reporter, "I learned early to drink beer, wine, whiskey, and I think I was about five when I first chewed tobacco." As an adult, he was an inveterate cigar smoker.

Today, the association between tobacco smoking and cancer of the larynx is well-established, but the role of alcohol in this disease is still debated. That being said, people who are exposed to secondary smoke and who also drink alcohol regularly carry a significantly higher risk of laryngeal cancer compared to those who abstain from alcohol. Alcohol appears to augment the ill effects of tobacco smoke. People who both smoke and drink regularly suffer 20 percent more smoking related lung cancers than those who smoke but do not drink alcoholic beverages. In addition, chewing tobacco puts one at risk for cancer of the mouth. However, multiple biopsies of Ruth's mouth showed negative results for cancer.

Babe Ruth died on August 16, 1948, in Memorial Hospital (now the Memorial Sloan Kettering Cancer Center) in Manhattan, where I served a fellowship in medical oncology 22 years later. An autopsy revealed he did not have cancer of the larynx. Rather, his cancer started in cells lining the upper part of the nasopharynx (the portion of the throat above the rear of the roof of the mouth and behind the nose). The cancer then spread by direct extension into the base of the skull, surrounding the cranial nerves, followed by local invasion into the left neck. There, the tumor surrounded the external carotid artery while metastasizing regionally by way of the lymphatic vessels into the lymph nodes. Ultimately, the malignancy traveled through the bloodstream into one lung, the liver and both adrenal glands—known as distant metastasis. Thus, Ruth's cancer used all three mechanisms at its disposal to wreak its havoc—direct invasion and metastasis through both the lymphatic vessels and blood vessels.

Because the nasopharynx lies above the roof of the mouth, it cannot be seen through the open mouth. It communicates with the cavity of the nose. Each of the nasopharynx's sidewalls contains an opening of the tube that leads to the middle ear—the Eustachian tube. The ceiling of the nasopharynx is the base of the skull. Today, clinicians use special instruments called endoscopes in a procedure called nasopharyngoscopy to visualize this hidden area, which was almost impossible to see with the equipment available in the 1940s.

Nasopharyngeal cancer is rare in the United States, representing less than 1 percent of all cancers. However, it is common in southern China, Southeast Asia, North Africa and the Middle East. For example, 25 of every 1,000 men in Hong Kong have this type of cancer, compared to only 0.5 of every 1,000 men in Connecticut. Most studies investigating a possible association between nasopharyngeal cancer and tobacco smoking have been carried out in high-risk populations, such as those in Asia, and have found no such association. In the low-risk United States, however, five studies have found an excess of nasopharyngeal cancer among smokers, with as much as a 6-fold higher risk in heavy smokers than in nonsmokers. This discrepancy in findings can be attributed to differences in the type of nasopharyngeal cancer that tends to occur in low-risk regions vs. high-risk regions.

The World Health Organization classifies nasopharyngeal cancer into two main types: non-keratinizing carcinoma and keratinizing squamous cell carcinoma. Non-keratinizing carcinoma accounts for 75 percent of nasopharyngeal cancers in the United States but more than 90percent in high-risk regions. For example, non-keratinizing carcinoma represents 99 percent of nasopharyngeal cancers in Hong Kong and is strongly associated with the Epstein-Barr virus, a type of herpes virus that also causes infectious mononucleosis. This virus is widespread and can cause mononucleosis in some people, typically in youth. The virus then becomes dormant inside the body but can become reactivated later in life. The virus is thought to play a role in the development of non-keratinizing carcinoma in certain susceptible ethnic and racial groups for unknown reasons. An interaction between particular genetic and environmental factors may be responsible.

Keratinizing squamous cell carcinoma accounts for about 25 percent of nasopharyngeal cancers in the United States, compared to 1 percent or fewer of such cancers in Hong Kong. It has only a weak association with the Epstein-Barr virus but a strong association with tobacco smoking. In regard to alcohol, studies have found a 33 percent-increased risk of all types of nasopharyngeal cancer among heavy drinkers. Some studies suggest keratinizing squamous cell carcinoma may not be as sensitive to irradiation treatment as non-keratinizing nasopharyngeal cancer. Furthermore, these studies indicate individuals with keratinizing squamous cell carcinoma may have a somewhat poorer 5-year survival rate than individuals with non-keratinizing nasopharyngeal cancer. Babe Ruth had keratinizing squamous cell carcinoma of the nasopharynx.

Why was Babe Ruth hoarse if there was no tumor in his larynx? What accounted for the initial symptoms that led to the misdiagnosis he had cancer of the larynx? The autopsy results on his body allow us to look through the retrospectroscope to establish the mechanism for the manifestations of his cancer.

The hoarseness and difficulty in swallowing was caused by a tumor that began growing at or near the left side of the roof of the nasopharynx, beneath the base of the skull. As this tumor increased in size, it put pressure on three cranial nerves that exit the skull through the left jugular foramen, an opening between the temporal and occipital bones, and the hypoglossal canal. The functions of these cranial nerves—designated as numbers 9 (glossopharyngeal nerve), 10 (vagus nerve), and 11 (spinal accessory nerve)—overlap to some extent. Not only do they control the muscles of speech, chewing and swallowing, but they also convey sensation from the tongue, mouth, throat and larynx. The tumor at this site led to Ruth's hoarseness, throat pain and difficulty swallowing, resulting in his weight loss.

The tumor quickly progressed to the middle portion of the skull base, encroaching on two branches of cranial nerve 5, the trigeminal nerve. The maxillary (upper jaw) branch of this nerve exits through the foramen rotundum in the sphenoid bone of the skull base, and its mandibular (lower jaw) branch exits through the foramen ovale of this bone. The trigeminal nerve has both sensory and motor functions. Its sensory fibers convey information on pain, temperature, touch and pressure from the eye, lower eyelid, nose, cheek, mouth, gums, teeth and front two-thirds of the tongue. The trigeminal nerve's motor fibers control the muscles of chewing. Encroachment of the tumor on the branches of this nerve probably accounted for Ruth's left eye pain, the swelling of the left side of his face, and his eating difficulties.

Babe Ruth benefited from both radiation and chemotherapy with a somewhat prolonged life, but relief of his symptoms was short-lived. We must be mindful that meaningful treatment modalities for cancer were developed in the post-World War II era and were in their infancy at the time of Ruth's illness. If Ruth received treatment today for his nasopharyngeal carcinoma, surgery would not typically be used as first-line treatment because of the deep and inaccessible location of the nasopharynx and its proximity to crucial nerve and blood vessel structures. Rather, he would receive a technique known as intensity modulated radiation therapy, which results in far fewer adverse effects than the radiation treatment used during the 1940s. Chemotherapy has also come a long way with the advent of more effective platinum-based drugs. It is now routine for chemotherapy and radiation to be used simultaneously in treating patients with Ruth's type of cancer.

Under our modern system of tumor staging, Babe Ruth's nasopharyngeal cancer would be diagnosed as a Stage-IVA cancer. Today, as a result of the increased efficacy of treatment for this disease, Ruth's chance of surviving for 5 years after diagnosis would be about 58 percent. Unfortunately, he survived only 2 years.

Nasopharyngeal cancer was difficult to diagnose in Babe Ruth's time, and it is still difficult to detect in an early, treatable stage. The nasopharynx is not easy to examine—as previously noted—and the symptoms of this cancer mimic those of many other conditions. Nevertheless, if a person notices any of the following symptoms, he or she should consult a physician:

• a lump in the neck caused by a swollen lymph nod

- blood in the saliva
- bloody discharge from the nose
- persistent nasal congestion
- hearing loss
- frequent ear infections
- frequent headaches

For more information on nasopharyngeal cancer—including symptoms, causes, risk factors, complications, diagnosis, treatment, coping and prevention—see the Mayo Clinic's website at www.mayoclinic.com/health/nasopharyngeal-carcinoma/DS00756.

A final thought: hindsight has 20/20 vision.

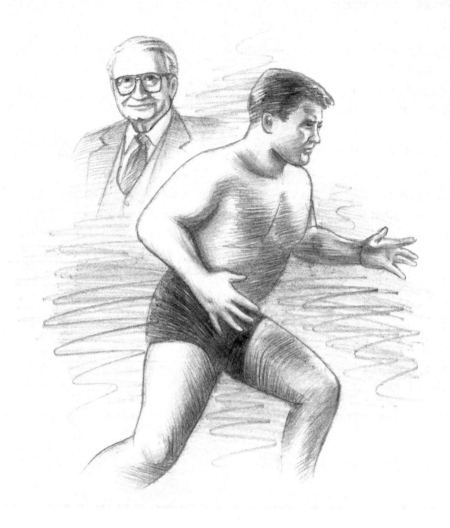

There had to be a Better Way

In July 1967, I was 28 years old and eager to begin a fellowship in hematology in the department of medicine at the University of Washington (UW) School of Medicine in Seattle. When I reported to the office of the Section of Hematology, a research assistant named Angela Bonica—a pretty brunette who appeared to be a few years younger than me—was assigned to give me a tour of the medical school and University Hospital. At the end of the tour, I asked Angela out on a date for the following Saturday night. She accepted but warned me her father was a strict, old-fashioned Italian who expected her to be home by midnight.

Following a movie, a tour of the city and a nightcap, I drove her home in time for her curfew. At about 11:55 p.m. we approached her house, which was on Mercer Island in the middle of Lake Washington. There must have been at least 10 cars in the long, winding driveway. I asked her if her folks were having a party. She said, "Oh, the WWWF must be in town. Those are my father's friends."

As a wrestling fan, I knew WWWF stood for World-Wide Wrestling Federation. I asked if her father was a professional wrestler. She laughed and replied, "Well, yes and no. Actually, he's chairman of the Department of Anesthesiology at UW, but he used to be a professional wrestler."

Absolutely intrigued, I asked Angela if I could meet her father. She responded by saying, "Of course. I'm sure he would be pleased that I had a date with an Italian," as if this was not a common occurrence. I accompanied her into the house.

Several large men, all wrestlers or former wrestlers—I recognized several—sat in the spacious living room. I was introduced to Gorgeous George (one of the most high-profile wrestlers in the world); Antonino Rocca (an Argentine who wrestled barefoot); Lou Thesz (one-time heavyweight champion); Johnny Valentine (the regional champ and local hero); Italian-born Bruno Sammartino; and many others, including Chief Little Wolf, Farmer Jones and Gypsy Joe. The names and faces of rest of the men are just blurs to me now.

Before I met these wrestlers, Angela introduced me to her father, John. He was a short, burly man with a prominent Roman nose, just like my father's. He shook my hand with an extraordinarily strong but disciplined grip, as if he was sending me a message—or so I thought.

John J. Bonica was born in 1917 on the idyllic island of Filicudi, one of the Aeolian Islands, about 20 to 30 miles northeast of Messina, Sicily. At age 11, he immigrated with his family to Brooklyn, New York, where he became the youngest (to this day) Eagle Scout from Brooklyn. A natural athlete, John took up wrestling, winning the New York City middleweight intercollegiate championship at the age of 17. Two years later, as a sophomore at Long Island University, he won the middleweight regional intercollegiate championship. After this bout, the nation's foremost wrestling promoter, Vince McMahon, Sr., convinced John to become a WWWF professional wrestler.

While wrestling professionally, John completed three years at Long Island University, followed by a year at New York University. He was an honor student who graduated with a bachelor of science degree in premedical studies. He wrestled in every major center in the Northeast and Midwest divisions of the WWWF. For four summers, John was also the strong man and wrestler for the Ringling Brothers and Barnum & Bailey Circus—the guy who "took on all comers." If you could last more than 10 minutes with him, you won a prize. No one ever won the prize.

In 1938, John entered the Marquette University School of Medicine in Milwaukee, Wisconsin, receiving his MD degree with honors in 1942. He was also inducted into the Alpha Omega Alpha Honor Medical Society, a professional medical organization that recognizes and advocates for excellence in scholarship. Incredibly, John continued to wrestle to support himself throughout his time in medical school. In 1938, he won the National USA title. A year later, he won the Canadian title, and in 1941, at age 24, he was light heavyweight champion of the world for seven months. He won these titles under the name Johnny "Bull" Walker. In Milwaukee, he wrestled as Joe Bucha to hide his identity from medical school officials, whom he feared might take a dim view of his extracurricular sporting activities.

Immediately after graduation, John married Emma Baldetti, whom he had met six years before when she attended one of his matches in Connecticut. John did a wartime-accelerated internship for six months, followed by 18 months of residency in anesthesiology at St. Vincent's Hospital in Manhattan. During his residency, Emma was in labor with Angela. In those days, a natural delivery was encouraged by most obstetricians—most of whom were men. It was customary that if a woman in labor received any anesthetic beyond a local, the anesthetic was ether dripped onto a mask placed over her mouth and nose. The ether rendered the woman unconscious. An inexperienced intern administered the drip ether to Emma. During the procedure, Emma began vomiting and choking on her stomach contents, causing her to gasp for air and turn blue. Dr. Bonica took control of the situation. He placed an endotracheal (breathing) tube into his wife's windpipe and connected the tube to a bag, which he squeezed 18 to 20 times a minute—essentially breathing for her. He undoubtedly saved the life of both his wife and child.

The experience caused Dr. Bonica to think there had to be a better way. It was this personal event that inspired him to initiate a campaign within the medical profession to improve obstetric pain relief and anesthesia during childbirth.

Dr. Bonica ultimately developed and initiated the use of epidural and caudal anesthetic techniques for women in labor, known today as conduction anesthesia. Thanks to these techniques, pain is eliminated while contractions of the uterus are preserved, as are movements of the limbs. The woman can remain awake during delivery, because the anesthetic is introduced around the covering of the spinal cord through a needle inserted into the lower back.

In 1944, at age 27, Dr. Bonica was inducted into the Army and assigned to Madigan Army Hospital at Fort Lewis in Tacoma, Washington. Madigan was the largest debarkation hospital of all the Armed Forces, receiving thousands of military personnel who had been wounded in the Pacific theater of World War II. He was made chief of anesthesiology with the rank of major.

His experiences at Madigan in treating patients with the pain of war wounds led Dr. Bonica to refine regional anesthesia techniques with the use of anesthetic agents applied to specific nerves. He clarified differences between treating patients with acute pain versus patients with chronic pain. Dr. Bonica introduced the concept of a multidisciplinary, team-based approach to the treatment of patients with pain—an approach that used the unique perspectives and expertise of neurologists, neurosurgeons, psychiatrists, surgeons and internists.

During his three years at Madigan, Dr. Bonica continued to wrestle professionally. Eventually, his commanding officer called him on the carpet, telling John his wrestling activities were conduct unbecoming of an officer—and forbidding John from wrestling publicly. But John did find a way to continue wrestling (more on that later).

Following his discharge from the Army, Dr. Bonica remained in Tacoma, as the chief of anesthesiology at Tacoma General Hospital. When Emma gave birth to their second daughter, Charlotte, she became the first woman in the Northwest to receive an epidural anesthetic during childbirth. The epidural was administered by an anesthesiologist trained by Dr. Bonica. John's experiences in the Army made him appreciate the advantages of using regional anesthesia, and he became an advocate for its use in surgical and obstetrical practices. The advantages of regional anesthesia extend to pain associated with invasive diagnostic procedures or surgery, as well as pain caused by such medical conditions as nerve compression resulting from cancer.

Dr. Bonica was inspired to conduct a systematic clinical study of pain syndromes and their treatment, and he continued to refine the multidisciplinary approach to pain management. He introduced the clinical concept that a patient's pain is influenced by what the patient feels and thinks it is, arguing the contemporary representation of pain excluded the influence of the mind. He called for adequate dosing of medications to prevent recurrent pain, rather than merely treating the pain after it recurred. Such dosing avoids the problem of the patient receiving too little too late with peaks and valleys in pain relief.

The doctor continued to wrestle regionally, despite the hospital administration and local medical society considering it unseemly for a physician to engage in the spectacle of professional wrestling. He disguised himself so he could wrestle without censure until 1950—when he finally ended a 15-year career as a professional wrestler of considerable repute.

In 1953, Dr. Bonica presented his innovative medical ideas in the first modern textbook of pain management, *The Management of Pain: With Special Emphasis on the Use of Analgesic Block in Diagnosis, Prognosis, and Therapy.* In what was to become the bible of pain diagnosis and treatment, JJB (as he was affectionately called by his peers) unfolded a new approach to pain as "neither exclusively physiologic, in which reaction, sensation, and intensity of the stimulus are all independent, nor subjective, in which perception and emotion are all important. Rather, pain is a dual phenomenon of reaction and perception." He argued that the perception of pain "involves the highest cognitive functions. It is what the individual feels, thinks, and does about the pain he possesses. Clinical action has to be based on the words and account of the patient in intractable pain." In the book, he championed "the recognition of pain as a disease, in and of itself, not merely a symptom of some other pathological condition." This revolutionary approach is as valid today as it was 60 years ago.

In 1956 and 1957, Dr. Bonica worked with Pope Pius XII on drafting the statement, "Man retains the right of control over the forces of nature. The Christian is never obliged to will suffering for its own sake. The doctor is seeking, in accordance with the ordinance of the Creator, to bring human suffering under man's control." Keep in mind that this statement was written at a time when many clergy still felt it was divine will to let nature takes its painful course in childbirth, and when cancer patients were encouraged to endure "redemptive suffering." I suspect Dr. Bonica had a hand in changing the pope's mind.

In 1960, Dr. Bonica was asked to be the founder and first chairman of the department of anesthesiology at the UW School of Medicine. For the next 18 years, he built the department into what many believed was the premier research, teaching and clinical standard of the world. The advances in regional anesthesia in surgery and obstetrics he initiated culminated in the 1967 publication of his classic text, "Obstetric Analgesia and Anesthesia: A Manual for Medical Students, Physicians in Training, Midwives, Nurses, and Other Health Personnel." That was also the year I first met the doctor. This book revolutionized obstetric care. It was updated in 1994 with contributions from multiple authors, and it remains the definitive reference in the field of obstetrics.

Following his visit to the People's Republic of China in 1972, President Richard Nixon directed the National Institutes of Health (NIH) to evaluate acupuncture and anesthesia as practiced in that country. Dr. Bonica was appointed chairman of the ad hoc committee on acupuncture of the NIH and a similar committee of American Society of Anesthesiologists. In 1973, he and 15 other members of the first official American medical delegation to visit China toured medical schools, hospitals and a variety of other health care facilities interviewing surgeons, anesthesiologists and scientists doing research on acupuncture anesthesia. Bonica reported the development and current status of acupuncture anesthesia in China and described its efficacy and clinical applications, suggesting its possible role in American medicine. In 1997, the NIH formally recognized acupuncture as a mainstream medicine healing option.

During his lifetime, Dr. Bonica authored or edited 41 books, was a collaborator and contributor to 60 other books, and wrote almost 300 scientific articles, two-thirds of which involved pain research and treatment. He died of a cerebral hemorrhage on August 15, 1994, at the age of 77.

And now for the rest of the story, as Paul Harvey used to say. This very high-profile immigrant, who typified the American Dream, served as a respected consultant to a U.S. president, fellow professors and even the pope. Why did he continue to wrestle well beyond any financial need? To hear him tell it, the reason was to "maintain my physical fitness and, especially, because I was good at it."

How did he continue to wrestle professionally after having been ordered to stop during his three years in the Army and during another three years at Tacoma General? It was with the help of his wife, Emma. She created a hood with two holes for the eyes and one for the mouth that he wore in the ring. Dr. Bonica was the professional wrestler whom you may have heard of as the Masked Marvel.

Some final thoughts: The Golden Age of wrestling began in the post-World War II period with the advent of television. The colorful and unforgettable characters were brought into the homes of millions of Americans as the TV craze swept the country as these professional athletes displayed their flamboyant and unique styles. A video clip from the '50s, still available on the Internet, featured Gorgeous George wearing a cape with gold bobby pins in his golden ringlets. He faced the short, burly Masked Marvel from Montana in the Seattle Aquatheater (www.youtube.com/watch?v=RB5VmdDmQ3M).

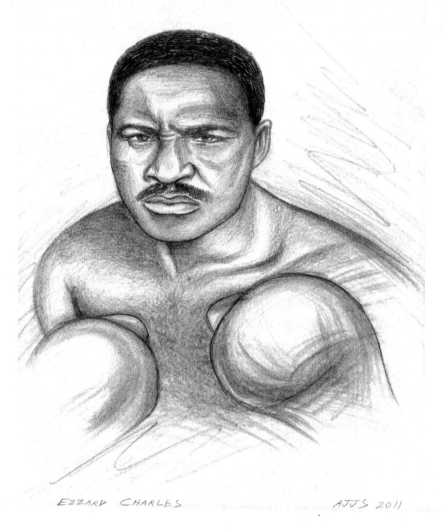

EZZARD CHARLES   AJJS 2011

Detroit Never Forgave Him

In the spring of 1965 in Hyde Park on the south side of Chicago, I
was a student doctor awaiting assignment to the next new patient in
the outpatient clinic of the Chicago Osteopathic Hospital. Louise,
the registrar, may have been unaware of the identity of the man
whose registration forms she had just put together. Or perhaps she
did know, because she gave me a sly wink as she handed me the
patient's chart. A compact woman with short black hair prematurely
streaked with gray, Louise's strong voice was gravelly from years of

two to three packs of cigarettes a day. My mother's age (in her mid-50s), she treated me as one of her favorites from the moment I told her my mother's name was also Louise. Whenever I greeted her, I would sing the verse of the old song that went, "Every little breeze seems to whisper Louise." When a new patient was to be assigned, she would bellow, "Next," into the anteroom where the slightly apprehensive, if not downright nervous, students awaited their turn. But not for me. She always preceded my last name with doctor, which was flattering yet intimidating because it reminded me of my awesome responsibility to the patient.

I glanced at the name on his chart, and called it out to a large waiting room filled with patients—some were new patients, others were waiting to be seen for follow-up and for consultation in the specialty clinics. A large, muscular black man sat in the far right corner with a child on each knee and several more at his feet. The children were apparently with other patients in the room, but they were visiting with and being entertained by this big man. When I called his name, he said a few words to the kids, who then scattered back to the people who they came with.

With considerable difficulty, he struggled to stand by using his huge arms for assistance and reached for his crutches. As he dragged himself toward the elevator door where I stood, I noticed he had a left foot drop and a slapping gait. He mentioned he was glad an elevator took us to the second floor examining rooms since he had difficulty climbing stairs.

While I was taking the patient's medical history, he said he worked as the athletic director for the South Side Chicago Park District, where he supervised the sports coaches. In a lower voice, he added that his main source of income was a liquor store. I believe he said it was on 85th Street about 30 blocks south. Almost reluctantly, he admitted he had been a professional boxer from 1940 to his retirement in 1959 (just 6 years prior to our meeting). In describing his symptoms, he told me he had difficulty with balance.

Upon physical examination, I detected muscle wasting and abnormal reflexes in his right lower leg. A detailed musculoskeletal examination revealed several areas of tissue texture abnormalities, lack of symmetry, restriction of joint motion and tender spots.

I presented the patient's case to the clinic supervisor, Dr. Kappler, who verified my findings with his own neurologic and structural examination. He instructed me to arrange for a consultation in neurology clinic, where I accompanied the patient and presented his case. The neurologist made a diagnosis of amyotrophic lateral sclerosis (ALS, commonly called Lou Gehrig's disease). The muscle wasting characteristic of this disease started in the patient's lower extremities rather than his upper extremities, which is more common. The neurologist suggested I seek further consultation in the osteopathic manipulative therapy (OMT) clinic to determine whether a course of OMT would improve his mobility. OMT techniques are designed to realign impaired joints by manipulation to relieve pain and tenderness and to improve function. They are based on the principles that the body as a whole, its structure and function are inter-related and inter-dependent. Consequently, musculoskeletal alignment can enhance and misalignment can impede function not only of the musculoskeletal system but of the nervous system and the organs served by the nervous system.
I treated the patient with OMT over the next three months. Seeing him on almost a weekly basis during that time, I got to know a quiet, unassuming and intelligent man. He was charismatic and exuded an aura of subtle greatness. There would always be children gathered around him in the waiting room as he, undoubtedly, told them stories about the benefits of discipline and training for sports and the virtues of being an athlete.

When I left for a hospital rotation in Detroit where I stayed for my internship, another student doctor continued treating him with OMT. Both the patient and I felt the treatment sessions were responsible for the definite improvement in his mobility to the point he could get by with a cane rather than crutches. However, I did not expect OMT would have any impact on the course of his ALS.

Flash forward 10 years. I took my family to the Mountain Shadows Resort and Golf Club in Scottsdale, Arizona, where I attended a medical seminar coincidentally entitled "Neurology for the Non-neurologist." The trip gave us an opportunity to visit my wife's 85-year-old great uncle, Nick Florio, and his wife Beth. The couple had retired to Sun City, and I was meeting them for the first time. Nick and his brother, Dan Florio, had been professional boxing trainers for Floyd Patterson, Jersey Joe Wolcott and dozens of well-known boxers from the 1940s through the 1960s. While driving to the home of Nick and Beth on May 28, 1975, we heard on the car radio that the boxer who was my patient when I was a student doctor had passed away from ALS at the age of 53. I could not wait to ask Nick if he knew him.

When I asked Nick about my former patient, his eyes lit up. With unexpected emotion and animation, he began to recount in great detail the fascinating highlights of the man whom I had never heard of until seeing him in the clinic.

Nick recalled, "In June 1949, he beat my own fighter, Jersey Joe Wolcott, on a 15 round decision in Chicago to win the national boxing championship. Then in 1950, he became world champion in Detroit with a 15 round decision over Joe Louis. He defended his title three times, but lost it in '51 in Pittsburgh to Joe Wolcott by a knockout in the 7th round. He got two more shots at the title, both against Rocky Marciano in '54. He lost the first on a 15 round decision that Marciano later said was the toughest fight he ever fought. He lost the second by a knockout. But he was the only one to last 15 rounds with Rocky Marciano!"

Then, with tears welling up in his eyes, Nick added, "You know, Detroit never forgave him for defeating Joe Louis. They felt that the only one who could or should be allowed to beat Louis would be a dynamic power hitter who dominated the sport. Instead, what they got was a champion (which Nick, as a native New Yorker, pronounced champeen) who feinted, countered, slipped and jabbed. He was too subtle to capture their imagination. The public wanted a more colorful, dominating presence in the ring and they just couldn't appreciate the subtle brilliance of his performances. Not only that but they felt that he was holding back in some of his most important bouts…that he was overly cautious. Well, do you want to know why?" I was riveted.

Nick continued, "He KO'd Archie Moore, a great fighter and future heavyweight champion, in January of '48. Six weeks later, he knocked out a tough young boxer named Sam Baroudi. Baroudi died of the injuries he sustained in that fight. He was so devastated by the death that he strongly considered getting out of the fight game. Afterwards, he adopted a more cautious style. He tried not to hurt his opponents. That is why he held back in some bouts."

That man, who had once been my patient-and the heavyweight boxing champion of the world, was Ezzard Charles, known in his prime as the Cincinnati Cobra. He battled ALS for 10 years, an unusually long course for this disease. I suspect his natural-born athleticism, fitness and training were the major contributors to his longevity but cannot help but think the OMT may have also played a role.

A final thought: Like life itself, boxing is the one sport in which, unless you are knocked out, neither the spectators nor the participants know the score or leader until the contest ends.

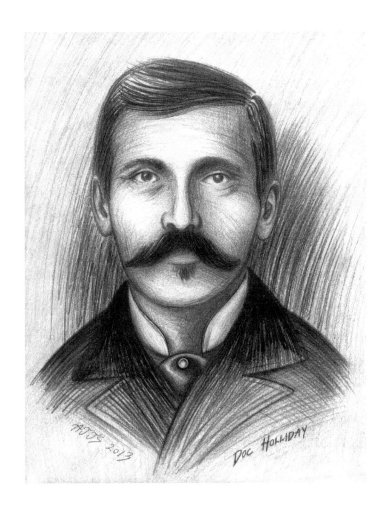

The Deadly Dentist

"He could be the poster child for a person with a chronic disease that eventually causes intractable pain and knows that he has a short time to live," was the description used by Dr. Forest Tennant, editor-in-chief of the medical journal, *Practical Pain Management.*

John Henry was born into a well-educated Southern family on August 14, 1851, in the town of Griffin, Georgia—now part of the Atlanta metropolitan area. While still a boy, his uncle John, a physician, gave him an 1851 Colt revolver to commemorate his birth year. The boy dedicated himself to becoming an expert marksman.

John's father, Henry, was a pharmacist and professional soldier with the rank of major. He participated in the Mexican War (1846-1848) and the War Between the States (Civil War) (1861-1865) for the South. Henry was away for most of John's childhood, resulting in the boy becoming much closer to his mother, Alice. She taught him to play the piano.

Before John was born, the major had brought home an orphaned Mexican boy, Francisco Hidalgo, when he returned from the Mexican War. Francisco became John's adopted brother.

When John was six years old, his father inherited land in Valdosta, Georgia, where the family of four moved. John was educated in the classics as well as math and science at Valdosta Institute, a school for Southern gentlemen. He studied Latin and Greek and became fluent in French.

John's mother died of tuberculosis (TB) in 1866 when he was 12. His adopted brother died of TB a short time later. John's father remarried three months after his wife's death.

Soon after these tragic personal losses, John moved into the home of his uncle, John Stiles Holliday, MD. There, a young, biracial servant named Sophie Walton taught him how to play card games called "Up and Down the River" and "Put and Take," which were similar to the card game, faro. Popular with Europeans in the 18th century, faro spread to the United States in the 19th century. It is played between a banker and several players, who win or lose according to whether cards the player turns up from a deck match or don't match cards already turned up. The games afforded John the opportunity, under Sophie's instruction, to learn how to count the cards in the deadwood (discarded pile) and to remember which cards were not played. John's competitive spirit, mathematical ability and excellent memory served him well when it came to playing cards.

John entered the Pennsylvania College of Dental Surgery at the age of 19. His choice of profession was probably encouraged by his cousin, Robert, who had founded the college. John graduated on March 1, 1872—five months before his 21st birthday. This was problematic because, in the state of Pennsylvania, one had to be 21 before receiving the Doctor of Dental Surgery (DDS) degree and being allowed to practice dentistry. For that reason, John served a student preceptorship under a classmate in St. Louis, Missouri, for five months before returning to Atlanta to begin his career as a licensed dentist.

At the age of 21—six months into his practice and nine years after his mother's death—Dr. John Henry Holliday began to lose weight. He attributed the weight loss to an active schedule. A hacking cough soon followed. He was diagnosed by his uncle John as having TB of the lungs. At that time, this condition was called consumption (weight loss) or phthisis (Greek for wasting). It was the same disease that had claimed the lives of his mother and stepbrother nine years earlier.

Dr. John Stiles Holliday told his nephew he likely had only six months to live. But he would be able to extend that time to two years if he moved to a warm, dry climate out West, ate a nutritious diet, consumed alcohol only in moderation, and enjoyed a prolonged rest. He followed only one of these recommendations.

On a hot and humid Atlanta day in September 1873, the dentist boarded a Western and Atlantic Railroad train with a one-way ticket to Dallas, Texas—the end of the line at that time. He was met by his new partner in dental practice, Dr. John A. Seegar. After settling in Dallas, John's consumption began to take its toll in the form of coughing episodes and periods of depression. His practice suffered because of frequent breaks and incessant coughing, which must have been disconcerting to his patients, especially during delicate dental procedures. He was forced to find another way to make a living. He started to spend time in gambling saloons and found his gambling more profitable than his dental practice had been.

Dr. John Henry Holliday's friends and gambling associates gave him the nickname "Doc." The name stuck. Doc was a natural at gambling, especially at playing poker and dealing faro. He also soon developed a reputation as a deadly gunfighter. The weak and frail dentist knew the Western frontier was a dangerous place for professional gamblers. The losing players were armed and often drunk and ready to fight. Doc honed his skills with both a six-shooter and a formidable-looking knife. But despite his reputation as a deadly gunman, Doc Holliday engaged in only eight shootouts during his lifetime. Of these, only two deaths have been verified. A third casualty of Doc's fighting fell victim to his knife. He had a remarkably fearless attitude toward death and danger. Perhaps it was because he was aware of his impending death from TB.

Tuberculosis was recognized as a contagious disease by the time of Hippocrates in 400 BC. However, it was not until 1882—10 years after the onset of active disease in John—that the responsible bacterium, mycobacterium tuberculosis, was isolated by the German physician, Robert Koch. This particular bacterium is a rod-shaped microbe known as a bacillus (plural, bacilli).

The natural history and biology of TB begins with small, airborne droplets of tuberculosis bacteria that are spread through the air when a person with active TB coughs or sneezes. If a person breathes in these germs and they become deposited in the lungs, there are four possible outcomes.

In some cases, the person's immune system is able to remove the bacteria, and he or she will not become ill.

In 5 percent of people exposed to TB bacteria, a rapidly progressive primary disease develops within two years of infection—typically within 6 to 18 months. The lungs are the most common site of active disease, known as TB pneumonia. The lymph nodes draining the area of infection enlarge in people with primary infection. In the absence of treatment, death ensues in 80percent of cases within about three years of infection (two years in the 19th century). In the remaining 20 percent of active disease cases, a chronic (long-term) condition develops, or the patient may recover. Chronic disease involves repeated episodes of scar tissue formation around the bacilli—an attempt by the body to contain the germs. The scar tissue repeatedly breaks down and reforms in a continuous cycle. Complete spontaneous eradication of the TB microbes in the setting of chronic TB is rare.

In 90 percent of exposed individuals, their natural immune response controls the bacteria by walling them off, causing the bacilli to be become dormant (inactive). This is called latent (hidden) infection. During this latent stage of TB infection, the individual is healthy and cannot spread the infection to others. It has been demonstrated that successfully contained latent TB confers immunity (protection) against subsequent TB infection. People who have had latent TB have a 79 percent lower risk of progressive TB following re-exposure to the germs, compared with people e not previously infected.

There is continued debate among experts regarding whether latent infection is able to become active disease more than five years after it has been acquired. It is possible the bacilli are no longer viable many years after infection, or the person's immune response is able to prevent living bacilli from reactivating and leading to disease. Many experts believe the development of active disease beyond five years after initial exposure is most often due to reinfection with new TB germs rather than reactivation of latent TB.

Among individuals with latent infection, reactivation of the disease will occur in 5 percent to 10 percent of cases. This reactivation differs from primary disease in that it tends to be localized to the upper rear portion of the lungs, with little lymph gland involvement.

Reactivation of latent TB results from growth of the dormant bacteria seeded at the time of initial infection. Reactivation TB may remain undiagnosed and potentially infectious for weeks, months or longer. Symptoms of reactivation begin slowly, with cough, weight loss and fatigue. Fever and night sweats are experienced by half the individuals afflicted with reactivation TB, along with chest pain, difficult breathing and blood in their sputum. Painful ulcers of the mouth, tongue, throat, stomach and intestines are caused by repeated coughing up and swallowing of highly infectious secretions. In the disease's advanced stages, loss of appetite, wasting (consumption) and malaise are experienced.

Bob Boze Bell, executive editor of True West Magazine and an historian and prolific writer about the Old West, provides a medically accurate description of TB in his book, *The Illustrated Life and Times of Doc Holliday*:

"Consumption can go undetected for some good time, especially if the tendency towards denial is followed. Fatigue is more and more pronounced as one's appetite seems to disappear. One feels 'out of sorts' and clammy. Periods of fever come and go. One wakes up in the dead of night drenched in sweat. In the morning, choking, coughing, and spitting up, at first watery fluid, later blood and chunks of lung tissue, rack the sufferer. The chest feels as if it was imploding and the pain of it all leads many to alcohol for temporary respite. To crown it all, many thought the illness a result of moral laxity. Compounded with terror of contagion, the consumptive becomes something of a pariah—a 'lunger' despised in and for his infirmity."

In a more modern description of the effects of TB, pain from the disease is caused by pressure placed on the left and/or right phrenic nerves by scar tissue or by direct invasion of bacteria. These nerves provide a dual function of controlling movement of the diaphragm as well as sensation to the diaphragm's central tendon and to the pericardium (sac covering of the heart) and the blood vessels of the chest. The disease process may also encroach on the intercostal nerves, found between the ribs. These nerves, in addition to their role in contracting the muscles of the rib cage, also register pain from the skin and lining of the rib cage. This nerve connection explains why damage to the internal wall of the chest can be felt as a sharp pain localized to the injured region.

In the final analysis, once infected with TB bacteria, active TB will develop in 10 percent to 15 percent of "normal" individuals during their lifetimes. There is a much greater chance of the disease developing in individuals with impaired immunity, such as those with HIV infection (who have 9-16 times the normal risk); those using high-dose cortisone-like drugs for a month or more; those using biologic agents as treatment for rheumatic diseases and inflammatory bowel disease; and those who have undergone kidney, heart, liver or allogeneic bone marrow or stem cell transplants. The antirejection drugs given to patients who have undergone such transplants suppress their immune systems, allowing the TB bacilli to become active.

Today in industrially developed countries, the rate of TB among the elderly is higher than among young adults, reflecting reactivation disease possibly attributed to impaired immunity associated with aging. But what about the situation in the Western frontier during the 1800s? The Old West can be thought of as a developing country. In third-world countries today, TB rates are highest among young adults, reflecting primary disease in this age group.

In the United States TB from recent infection has been shown to be seasonal, with a peak in the spring and a low occurrence in the autumn. Reactivation tuberculosis does not have a seasonal pattern.

The rate of TB is higher among men than women, beginning in the young adult years and persisting throughout life. This long-standing observation, dating back hundreds of years, is thought to reflect more frequent TB exposure among men than women rather than gender related.

The risk of active TB, whether of the primary or reactivation type, is substantially elevated in individuals who consume more than one daily shot—1.5 ounces (42 grams) of whiskey. This increased risk may be the result of the effects of alcohol on the immune system. There are no reports that Doc Holliday drank alcohol to excess, if at all, prior to the advent of his TB. However, there are several references to him being an alcoholic subsequent to the diagnosis of TB.

Cigarette smoking confers a 1.5 to 2 times greater chance of the development of TB. Smoking has also been associated with the risk of relapse and death from TB. Passive (second-hand) smoking also increases the risk for TB. Historians have provided us with no information regarding Dr. Holliday's smoking habits. But there is no doubt, based on his lifestyle, that he was exposed to second-hand smoke from ages 22 to 36. During that period of his life, he frequented saloons, gambling halls and houses of prostitution.

The most important risk factor for TB of the lungs is close household contact with an individual who has the disease. Historians generally believe John Holliday and his brother Francisco contracted TB from their mother. This route of disease transmission was probably true for Francisco, but was it also true for John? Based on the preceding portrayal of the natural history and epidemiology of TB, one could make the case for three possible scenarios. You be the judge.

If John and Francisco contracted primary TB from their mother, we might assume the mother developed active TB two years prior to her death, when John was 12 years old. In my opinion, that is the least likely scenario, because the incubation period in John—from initial contact with his infective mother to the expression of an active, acute phase of the disease—would have been a minimum of

9 years and a maximum of 11 years. This time is inconsistent with what we know about untreated TB. Primary disease usually occurs within two years. Reactivation after nine or more years can occur, but it becomes progressively less common after five years.

It is possible Dr. Holliday was infected by one of his patients while in dental school or during his first year of practice. It is doubtful he took any precautions when treating a coughing patient who could potentially be transmitting the disease. This possibility would be consistent with primary disease developing within the usual two-year window following infection. Thus, that is the scenario I favor. Doctor Alexander Irwin, a dentist who practiced in Southfield, Michigan, for 62 years, recently related to me that when he started his dental practice, "tuberculosis was an occupational hazard for dentists." Effective treatment for patients with TB was not developed until 1952 with the introduction of Isoniazid (INH). The less effective agent streptomycin, a product of wartime research, became available in 1946 and para-aminosalicylic acid (PAS) soon after.

Failing a spontaneous cure, the doctor lapsed into chronic, progressive disease, from which he met his ultimate demise 15 to 17 years after becoming infected. Considering his lifestyle after the onset of his tuberculosis, it is inexplicable to me how or why he survived 13 to 15 years beyond the dire but realistic prognosis rendered by his uncle.

Doc used three medicinals in the treatment of his ailment—alcohol, opium and bugleweed.

Several writers have alluded to Doc being intoxicated. He is said to have drank as much as four quarts of whiskey a day. The alcohol apparently relieved his pain as well as erased his fear of death. However, Kate Elder, his longtime companion, consort and common-law wife, reportedly said, "He was not a drunkard. He always had a bottle of whiskey but never drank habitually. When he needed a drink, he would only take a small one." Could a person be inebriated on a regular basis if he was also alert enough to count cards and have enough manual dexterity to gamble professionally, use a gun and knife with accuracy, and ride a horse? More likely, Holliday used a daily maintenance dose of alcohol to suppress his cough and pain. I suspect he, as a formally trained healthcare professional, was adept at establishing the optimal dose and interval of alcohol intake. For a variety of reasons, with which we are all familiar, alcohol is difficult to titrate as if it were a pharmaceutical. No doubt, he occasionally overdosed.

As his condition deteriorated, Doc turned to the use of an opium preparation called laudanum. Today, it is known as tincture of opium. In the 1800s, opium was the standard treatment for patients with symptoms of TB. At that time, nearly all consumptives used some form of opium to quiet their cough, control their diarrhea, reduce their stress, and relieve their pain. The formulation Doc used was flavored with either cinnamon or saffron. It was sold without a prescription and was the main ingredient in the patent medicines of the 19th century. Opium is not pure. It contains small amounts of codeine, morphine and other opioids (compounds that reduce pain and cause a sense of euphoria).

Bugleweed is an herb in the mint family native to Europe. It was brought to the American colonies in the 1700s. The plant's botanical name, lycopus, refers to the resemblance of its cut leaf to a wolf's paw. This also accounts for various common names that, in many languages, refer to wolves. In English, it is sometimes referred to as green wolf's foot. The herb was traditionally used to make extracts and tinctures, primarily for reducing pain. Bugleweed also has sedative, astringent (causing contraction of tissues and reduction of bleeding), and mildly narcotic (causing insensibility or stupor) properties. Advocates for its use today claim it, "supports bronchial and respiratory passages and occasional nervous tension." In the 19th century, bugleweed was routinely used in treatment if the consumptive coughed up so much blood that a blood vessel ruptured and bled into the lungs.

Doc Holliday's main notoriety stems from his participation in the notorious Gunfight at the OK Corral, which took place in Tombstone, Arizona, on October 26, 1881. Lasting only 30 seconds, this gunfight has long captured the imagination and fascination of the American public. The personal appearance, behavior and demeanor of a man given a terminal prognosis and suffering from the ravages of a relentless disease have been immortalized in several books and Hollywood movies, with typical historical license.

The truth is Doc Holliday was a very intelligent and well-educated man. He was able to find his intellectual equal and happiness with Kate Elder, despite her checkered past as a prostitute and "sporting girl" who worked in saloons and gambling houses. The Hungarian-born daughter of a physician, she had an aristocratic education and spoke four languages, including French.

Kate reportedly painted this portrait of Doc:

"Doc was close to 6 feet tall, weighed 160 pounds, fair complexion, very pretty mustache, blue-grey eyes, and fine set of teeth. He never boasted of his fighting qualities. He was a neat dresser, and saw to it his wife was dressed as nicely as himself."

It must be said that Doc tried to maintain his dignity and sense of professionalism throughout his medical ordeal. The doctor was always smartly dressed, typically wearing a gray sport coat with a bow tie or a cravat fastened with a diamond stick-pin. A cravat, in those days, was a wide, straight scarf worn around an open-necked shirt. In contrast to an ascot, it is worked loosely and not tied (thereby requiring a stick-pin).

Another perspective about Doc can be gained from his friend and fellow participant in the Gunfight at the OK Corral, Wyatt Earp. In his memoirs, Earp wrote, "I found him a loyal friend and good company. He was a dentist whom necessity had made a frontier vagabond, a philosopher whom life had made a caustic wit, a long, lean, ash-blonde fellow nearly dead with consumption and at the same time the most skillful gambler and the nerviest, speediest, deadliest man with a six-gun I ever knew."

Wyatt Earp told a colorful tale about an incident that occurred in Fort Griffin, Texas. Doc Holliday was dealing cards to the town bully, Ed Bailey, who was not intimidated by Doc's reputation. In an ill-advised attempt to irritate Doc, Bailey kept picking up the discards and looking at them. This was a no-no according to the rules of Western poker and could result in forfeiting the pot. Holliday warned Bailey about this twice. When Bailey picked them up the third time, Doc raked in the pot without showing his hand or saying a word. Bailey began to raise his pistol from under the table. But before he could cock the hammer, Doc's large knife slashed across his abdomen, spilling his blood and guts onto the table.

Doc made no attempt to run from the scene, knowing his actions were in self-defense. Yet, he was arrested and held in a local hotel room under armed guard. When Kate Elder spotted a vigilante mob making its way to the hotel, she set fire to a shed, drawing the town's attention to the fire. While the townspeople were engaged in fighting the fire, Kate confronted the guard with a pistol in each hand and successfully disarmed him. She and Doc then escaped to Dodge City, Kansas, riding stolen horses. They registered at Deacon Cox's Boarding House as Dr. and Mrs. J. H. Holliday.

Doc so appreciated what Kate had done that, in an effort to please her, he made a short-lived attempt to return to the practice of dentistry. She, in turn, promised to give up her life of prostitution and frequenting saloons. Nether of their resolutions lasted during their on-again, off-again, turbulent relationship. In Doc Holliday's final days, Kate traveled to Glenwood Springs, Colorado, where she ministered to him and probably helped to support the destitute dentist, gambler and gun and knife fighter.

W.B. "Bat" Masterson wrote a series of articles about the gunman he knew when he was sheriff of Dodge City and Pueblo, Colorado. His first-person accounts were originally published in Human Life Magazine in 1907 and republished in book form in 1957 and again in 2009 under the title, *Famous Gunfighters of the Western Frontier.* One of Masterson's unflattering descriptions of Doc was that of "a weakling who could not have whipped a healthy 15-year-old boy in a go-as-you-please fistfight."

John C. Jacobs, a fellow gambler and casino operator, described Doc Holliday as a volatile man who had repeated episodes of intolerable pain as well as mood swings and hostile behaviors. He said of Doc:

"This fellow Holliday was a consumptive and a hard drinker, but neither liquor nor the bugs seem to faze him. He could at times be the most genteel, affable chap you ever saw, and at other times he was sour and surly, and would just as soon cut your throat with a villainous-looking knife he always carried, or shoot you with a 41-caliber double-barreled derringer he always kept in his vest pocket."

Historians agree Doc's health began to fail dramatically in 1884. While working as a faro dealer in Leadville, Colorado, he suffered severe weight loss, mental confusion, extreme fatigue and generalized weakness. Observers could see that as he deteriorated, Doc could no longer deal cards or work as a gambler. He visited the hot springs in Glenwood Springs, Colorado, hoping they might bring him some relief. But the sulfur fumes emanating from the springs may have done his lungs more harm than good.

Lapsing into a coma, Dr. John Holliday spent his final days in the Glenwood Hotel. One of the most famous victims of tuberculosis in United States history died on November 8, 1887, at the age of 36.

Some final thoughts: There are no reports of any of Doc Holliday's close friends or associates contracting tuberculosis from him. This includes Kate Elder, who lived to almost 90 years of age. Kate's 10-year affair with Doc began in the fall of 1877 after she first met him in a Fort Griffin saloon. According to Kate, who was with him when he died, Doc looked down at his bare feet while lying in bed and uttered his last words, "This is funny." Kate knew what those words meant. Doc always thought that he would die with his boots on. According to Old West folklore, if you died old and sick, you died with your boots off in bed. If you died in a gunfight or while gambling, you died with your boots on.

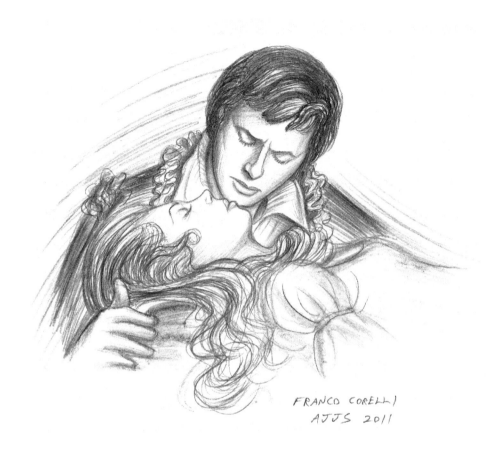

FRANCO CORELLI
AJJS 2011

He Could Not Read a Note

No one knew his first name. Mr. Milani managed the claque concession at the Metropolitan Opera House. The claque is a term derived from the French word meaning hand clap. It refers to a group of individuals hired to yell out the seemingly spontaneous bravos, bravas and bravis heard during an opera. One of their duties is to applaud at just the right moment to cue the audience an aria has ended—thereby avoiding the embarrassment of people clapping prematurely. Claque members are also the ardent admirers who are seen handing bouquets of flowers, with great flourish, to the divas as they take their bows at the finale.

While in college, I got a job at the old Met, on Broadway between 39th and 40th streets in New York City. My uncle Louis was the house physician there from 1950 to its close in 1966, when the Met was moved to Lincoln Center. He arranged for me to be a member of the claque, actually employed as needed by Mr. Milani for a unique service. I was to drive the Italian opera stars from Idlewild Airport (called John F. Kennedy International Airport since 1963) to the Roosevelt Hotel on Madison and 45th Street, where tradition dictated they stay during their performances. Because I was sufficiently fluent in Italian, I was comfortable with this plum job.

On one of my assignments, the star I picked up at the airport was the great Italian tenor Franco Corelli, who was 40 years old at the time. He insisted I put the top up on my black 1957 Ford Fairlane convertible, claiming the wind might affect his voice. Although the traffic on the Van Wyck Expressway was light in those days, his eyes darted nervously from lane to lane. Was it my youth? Was it my driving? Or was it a reflection of his personality? I tried not to take it personally. His command of the English language was decent, but he preferred to speak Italian in what little conversation there was between us during the drive to the hotel.

Corelli was a strikingly handsome but quirky man with a strong voice that had a phenomenal range. He was capable of a high, fast vibrato (not a tremolo) as well as a low baritone. However, he was very insecure and suffered from terrible stage fright. Before every performance, he swallowed a 20-milligram Valium tablet to relieve his anxiety (that high dose was available in Italy but not in the United States) and three cloves of garlic. Corelli believed the garlic protected his voice from cracking. I suspect the garlic strongly contributed to the swooning of the sopranos with whom he sang duets.

One cause of Corelli's insecurity—or at least his self-consciousness—may have been that he was bald in a business where looks are so highly valued. He always wore a hairpiece both on and off the stage. But the main reason for Corelli's insecurity was he sang by ear and could not read a note of music. In addition, he had little formal voice training. He essentially taught himself by mimicking the recorded voices and styles of the legendary opera greats from the previous generation—such tenors as Giacomo Lauri-Volpi, Enrico Caruso and Beniamino Gigli. Although most opera singers perform from memory, there were some real stars who could not read sheet music. *The King and I*—published in 2004 by one of Luciano Pavarotti's former managers, Herbert Breslin—is critical of Pavarotti's inability to read music. Pavarotti denied he could not read music in a 2005 interview with Jeremy Paxman on the BBC, but acknowledged he did not read orchestral scores. The same was said of Mario Lanza. Analogous to people with a learning disability, those who sing by ear compensate by studying with conductors whose tempo and interpretation of the orchestral scores is closest to their individual style-as they heard the music. In an interview with Stefan Zucker for the Opera News, Corelli was asked about a run-in with conductor Fabien Sevitzky during rehearsals for the opera *Carmen* at the opera house in Verona, Italy. He said about Sevitzky, "He was more interested in the design of the accompaniment than in the vocal lines and highlighted the orchestration at the expense of the singers. Some of his tempos were extremely fast, others unduly broad." The end result is a pairing between singer and orchestra conductor similar to what is done conventionally by pop singers. An example is the pairing of Frank Sinatra and Nelson Riddle.

In 1958, a boy was born in Tuscany with congenital glaucoma, an elevation of the pressure of fluid inside the eyes. He was rendered visually impaired despite multiple surgeries and the daily application of eye drops. With the prediction the young man would ultimately be blind he was enrolled in a boarding school where he was taught to read Braille. Andrea was a child prodigy who, at age six, began playing piano and several other instruments, including the flute and saxophone. At age 12, he suffered a blow to the head while tending goal during a soccer game. This resulted in hemorrhages into the occiput (the back part of the brain where sight registers) as a result of the soccer accident. Although there was no obvious damage to the eyes or the optic nerves, the hemorrhages left him completely blind from the brain damage. Andrea Bocelli adapted to his blindness and went on to study law at the University of Pisa, financing his education by singing in piano bars and nightclubs.

One night in 1992, the Italian rock star and blues artist known as Zucchero (his stage name means sugar in Italian) heard the 34-year-old Bocelli singing pop songs in a nightclub and was impressed with his voice. As the legend goes, he approached him and said something to the effect, "The quality and timbre of your voice tell me that you were meant to sing opera." Bocelli reportedly responded by asking, "What operatic voice coach would take me on? I'm blind and, obviously, I cannot read music." Zucchero probably said, "I know just the guy, and he could use the work."

Zucchero recruited 71-year-old Franco Corelli to be Bocelli's voice coach. Corelli had retired from the stage prematurely at age 55 in 1976 as an emotional wreck. In the same interview in the Opera News mentioned above, Corelli admitted "I was full of apprehension and mad at everyone. I was a bundle of nerves, I wasn't eating or sleeping."

It was a perfect match—Bocelli with a physical challenge to a vital organ, and Corelli with a disabling mental challenge. They were brought together by an instrument they both played by ear—their voice. Neither could read a note.

Thus began the meteoric rise of tenor Andrea Bocelli in the world of opera. Bocelli's eclectic musical background helps explain why the famous crossover star can sing not only "Nessun dorma" in Puccini's opera, *Turandot*, and "La donna è mobile" in Verdi's *Rigoletto*—but also such popular hits as "Con te partirò" ("Time to

Say Goodbye") with Sarah Brightman and "The Prayer" with Celine Dion.

A final thought: A quote from H.L. Mencken—"Opera in English is about as sensible as baseball in Italian."

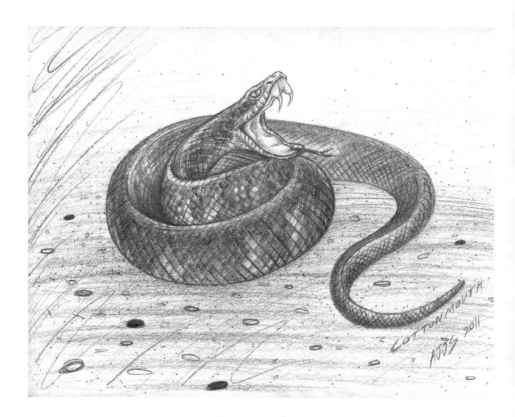

Snakebite!

As the priest at Holy Family Cathedral in Tulsa, Oklahoma, masterfully weaved his sermon toward its climax, he inserted a dramatic pause in the thunderous crescendo. At that precise moment, my Motorola audio pager went off. The voice of the hospital operator reverberated throughout the cavernous cathedral, loud and clear, with the message, "Dr. Perrotta! Dr. Perrotta! Emergency room! Stat! Snakebite victim!"

I leaped up from the pew and ran the length of the center aisle toward the large oak entry doors at the rear of the cathedral. In the background I heard scores of whispering voices, most likely exchanging their experiences with snakebites. The priest was speechless for what seemed like the entire time I was sprinting toward the exit. He must have been stunned that I had just destroyed his eloquent sermon, which had been delivered with the cadence and rhythm of a Southern evangelist, after whom it was undoubtedly modeled. After all, this was the Bible Belt, and he was competing for souls with the orations of such renowned preachers as Tulsa's healing evangelist, Oral Roberts.

It was May 1971, and I was a resident in internal medicine at Oklahoma Osteopathic Hospital in Tulsa. Dorothy, my wife of only six months, and I shared one car. During the week, she would drop me off at the hospital in the morning, proceed to the elementary school near the airport where she taught remedial reading, and pick me up in the evening. On the Sundays of weekends I was on duty as the on-call internal medicine resident, we would go to the 8 a.m. Mass at Holy Family Cathedral on 8th and Boulder, because it was closer to the hospital than our local church. The cathedral could easily seat 1,000 people, but there were no more than 60 in the pews that day my pager alarmed the congregation with the snakebite call.

I frantically responded to the call and hurriedly drove to the hospital, oblivious that I had left my wife at the Mass without any means of transportation. All I could think about was I didn't know a damn thing about snakebites. The only snakes I had ever seen were in the Reptile House at the Bronx Zoo when I was in grade school. Speeding toward the hospital, I desperately tried to recall what I had learned in medical school on the topic several years before. What I could remember would basically pass for first aid—an antivenin was available and there was a difference in the signs and symptoms of a pit viper bite versus a coral snake bite, with the latter being toxic to the nervous system. An antivenin is a serum containing an antitoxin designed to neutralize venom from snakes or other animals.

By the time I entered the emergency room (ER), my pulse must have been faster than that of the man in his thirties whom I found lying on a gurney with both legs elevated. The front of his very swollen and tense left shin shone with a purple glaze accentuating

45

two apparent puncture marks midway up the front of his shin bone oozing blood. He was sweaty and obviously very uncomfortable, his pulse rapid.

The ER physician was a laid-back good ol' boy, a native Oklahoman who looked and sounded to me like the cowboy actor, Randolph Scott. He was cool, calm and collected, and I sensed he had considerable experience with snakebite victims. Without any prompting on my part, he gave me a detailed rundown on the patient, probably sensing this city boy's apprehension and abject ignorance about the proper treatment for snakebites. He informed me the patient had no sensation between his great (first) toe and second toe, suggesting the man had an "anterior compartment syndrome" of the left leg. The doctor added that the patient was a ranch hand who was mucking out a cattle pond when he was bitten by a cottonmouth (whatever that was). Pit viper antivenin had been administered to the gentleman before my arrival.

Results of the patient's laboratory tests showed no signs of a clotting abnormality or kidney failure. I subsequently learned snake venom can destroy not only muscle tissue near the bite (a condition called necrosis), but also muscle tissue distant to the wound site (called rhabdomyolysis). As a result of this muscle breakdown, a muscle protein called myoglobin is released into the bloodstream. When myoglobin reaches the kidneys, it can cause kidney failure, requiring the patient to receive dialysis. The snake venom can also affect the clotting system in the bloodstream, leading to the breakdown of blood coagulation factors, which causes widespread bleeding unless these factors are replaced.

I was told the patient was to be admitted to an internal medicine service, which is why I was called. However, a surgical consultation had been requested to determine whether the patient was a candidate for fasciotomy, a surgical procedure in which fascia (the connective tissue around muscles) is cut away to relieve tension or pressure. The leg consists of four separate groups of muscles, arteries, veins and nerves. Each group is surrounded by an elastic sheath of fascia, forming a kind of compartment. The anterior (front) compartment contains the four extensor muscles of the foot (those muscles that lift the foot toward the shin), the anterior tibial artery, and the deep peroneal nerve.

I learned a venomous snakebite to the leg can cause a breakdown of muscle tissue and inflammation that leads to the accumulation of fluid (a condition called edema) within the leg's anterior compartment. The fascial covering prevents expansion of the compartment to compensate for the swelling. Known as anterior compartment syndrome, this condition is a rare complication of snakebites, even in a very swollen limb. Nevertheless, if left unchecked, it can result in pressure on the deep peroneal nerve, resulting in foot drop, claw foot and paralysis. This accumulating, trapped fluid also increases pressure on the easily compressible veins, thereby decreasing outflow of blood through those veins. Initially, the flow of blood though the arteries remains intact, so blood comes into the compartment but does not go out. This results in more swelling. The arterial blood supply can be lost when the pressure within the compartment becomes so intense the anterior tibial artery is compressed. The worst-case scenario is amputation of a limb that has lost its blood supply.

The definitive treatment for patients with anterior compartment syndrome involves cutting into the fascia on both sides of the compartment with a large incision through the skin and fascia. The incision releases the fluid and relieves the pressure.

As I was absorbing the information given to me by the ER doctor, the chief resident in surgery, another tall, lanky Oklahoman, entered the room. He looked at the patient's purple extremity and gently pushed the man's left foot toward his shin, eliciting an agonizing scream. The surgical resident turned to me and said, "If you give him medical clearance, I'll take him up to surgery right now. He has an acute anterior compartment syndrome that has to be decompressed right away, or he'll lose this leg. I can't feel any pulse, and that foot is as white as the sheet under him."

Having regained my composure, I replied in a quasi-authoritative tone, "Yes, he has medical clearance. I've reviewed his lab work with the ER doc, and he has no medical contraindications." The patient was then whisked up to the surgical suite.

I turned to the ER doctor and asked, "How did you know it was a cottonmouth?"

Instead of answering, he reached into a water basin that was on a stand near where the gurney had been. He carefully picked up something from within the basin, then turned and handed me a very dark—almost black—snake about four feet long. He seemed to enjoy my reaction as I jumped backward, wondering if the slimy serpent was still alive. It wasn't. The staff standing in the hallway was obviously tuned into the prank, based on the roar of laughter that erupted from the heads peeking through the doorway.

With latex-gloved hands, the prankster pried opened the dead snake's mouth to show me the white interior of its mouth and throat, noting, "Hence the name cottonmouth." At that point, I suddenly remembered I had left Dorothy at the cathedral. I figured I had enough time to pick her up while the patient was still in surgery. So I headed back to my car.

Dorothy had been waiting for me on the steps of the church for at least an hour, and I profusely apologized to her. I then shared my ER encounter with her. She had about as much prior experience with snakes as I did, since she also grew up in the Bronx and had encountered snakes only in the Bronx Zoo. Needless to say, she was horrified by my description of the unfortunate patient, and she must have been wondering why, in God's name, I had taken her away from her idyllic home in Pelham Manor, New York, and brought her to this land of snakes.

48

That day, I decided to learn all about the cottonmouths and other pit vipers of Oklahoma to help prepare me for future clinical encounters in the event I would be confronted with this situation again.

There are several species of venomous snakes in Oklahoma, including the cottonmouth (also called water moccasin), the copperhead, and five kinds of rattlesnakes (the prairie, timber, western diamondback, western massasauga and western pigmy rattlesnakes). All are members of the pit viper subfamily, Crotalinae, of the viper family, Viperidae. The term pit viper refers to the heat-sensing pit between the eye and nostril on each side of the head. This organ enables the snake to detect and strike warm-blooded prey, such as mice and birds, in total darkness. These snakes also eat such cold-blooded animals as fish, frogs and lizards.

Pit vipers and other snakes use their tongues to detect odors, by sticking the tongue out to pick up scent particles from the air or ground and then pulling the tongue back to deposit the particles in a sensitive organ in the roof of the mouth called Jacobson's organ. This organ enables a snake to recognize and follow the scent of its prey. Snakes can also detect vibrations in the ground and air to help them determine the size of available prey or approaching enemies.

The cottonmouth and copperhead are usually found in watery habitats, such as streams, rivers, lakes, marshes, swamps, sloughs, reservoirs, canals, retention pools, cattle ponds and even roadside ditches. The cottonmouth is one of the most common venomous snakes in Oklahoma, as well as the most aggressive pit viper in the state. Young cottonmouths have obvious reddish brown crossbands on their bodies, often with speckles and spots. This pattern darkens with age, so that adults may be almost uniformly dark black with a lighter underbelly. A distinguishing characteristic of cottonmouths is a dark streak on the side of the head that runs from the eye to just past the corner of the mouth. Adult cottonmouths typically range in length from about 20 to 48 inches (51 to 122 centimeters), though some have been known to grow as long as 6 feet (1.8 meters) or more.

The patient got struck by the cottonmouth as he was raking vegetation out of a pond used by cattle for drinking water on a ranch. Abundant plant and algal life growing in such ponds can cause periodic low oxygen levels in the water, so the ponds have to be regularly mucked out. As the ranch hand was engaged in this task, the snake, with half its body floating in the water, reared its fearsome head and bit him on the left shin, the tibial region. He managed to kill the serpent with his rake, and he brought the dead reptile to the hospital to show the doctors.

When threatened, the cottonmouth coils and opens its mouth wide, displaying its retractable hollow fangs and the white interior of its mouth. The snake's potentially deadly venom is released into the fangs from special glands under the reptile's control. Snakes can regulate whether to release venom, and how much venom to release, when they bite. That is why someone can be bitten by a cottonmouth but not necessarily be injected with its venom. So-called dry bites (in which no venom is injected) occur in an estimated 25 percent of pit viper bites. The cottonmouth is more likely to inject venom (a process called envenomation) when killing prey than when protecting itself from enemies. Cottonmouth envenomation typically causes less severe signs and symptoms than rattlesnake envenomation but more severe signs and symptoms than copperhead envenomation.

The pain from cottonmouth envenomation is generally described as more severe than that of its pit viper cousins. In the leg, such severe pain is an early and sensitive sign of anterior compartment syndrome—as in the case described.

Furthermore, there is usually more bleeding under the skin with cottonmouth envenomation than with other pit viper envenomation, but there is usually more fluid-filled blisters with rattlesnake envenomation than with that of cottonmouths.

The height of the snake season in Oklahoma is between April and October, peaking between July and August. The majority of all snakebites are to the lower extremities.

The patient was given a polyvalent antivenin that, in those days, was made from antibodies derived from the serum of a horse purposely exposed to the snake's venom. The term polyvalent refers to the fact the antivenin contains antibodies against the venom of multiple species of pit viper. Today, the antivenin used for pit viper bites is much more refined than it was in the 1970s, resulting in far fewer adverse reactions in patients. The antibodies used to make the antivenin are now obtained from sheep rather than from horse serum.

People living in regions where venomous snakes are common should be advised on how to recognize such snakes. In general, the following five features can help you identify a snake as venomous (modified from Bruce Peverly, *Poisonous Snakes of Oklahoma* www.tulsamastergardeners.org/snake/snakes.shtml accessed 10-25-2011.

The presence of rattles on the tail indicates the snake is venomous. Only rattlesnakes have rattles.

Except for coral snakes, venomous snakes in the United States tend to have triangular or diamond-shaped heads that are distinctly broader than their necks. Nonvenomous snakes, by contrast, have narrow heads that are typically only slightly wider than, or the same width as, their necks.

A depression (the pit) on the sides of the face between the eyes and nostrils identifies a pit viper.

Vertical eye pupils (so-called cat's eyes) are a strong indication a snake is venomous.

Venomous snakes have a single row of scales immediately behind the anus, while nonvenomous snakes typically have two rows of scales in that location.

The ranch hand's encounter with a venomous snake turned out well thanks to the timely and decisive action of the ER physician and the surgical resident. They had previous experience with the potential complications of pit viper bites, as well as the actual complication experienced by a grateful patient. The patient's leg was salvaged, and the incisions healed within two weeks. Fortunately, that ER experience was my only exposure to snakebite for the remainder of the year.

Six months later, I returned to New York to begin a fellowship in medical oncology at the Memorial Sloan-Kettering Cancer Center in Manhattan—where the Central Park Zoo now has one boa and several pythons but, thankfully, no pit vipers. I suspect they all have Medicare.

A final thought: "If you see a snake, just kill it—don't appoint a committee on snakes."—quote from Ross Perot

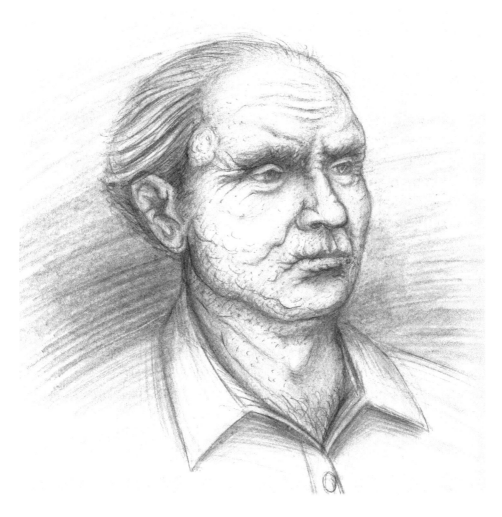

The Leper on the Bus

All 500 seats in the amphitheater within University Hospital, the teaching hospital of the University of Washington School Of Medicine in Seattle, were filled on this Saturday morning in the fall of 1967. The gathering was part of the Grand Rounds in Medicine, in which the most interesting, informative or challenging case of the month was presented by the chief resident in medicine, followed by an in-depth discussion of the case by the appropriate faculty member for the topic. By unwritten protocol, faculty professors and chiefs of the various medical specialties sat in front; house staff (students, interns, residents and fellows) in the rear; and community practitioners in the middle. As a fellow, I was sitting a few rows from the back. It was standing-room only on this day.

Unusual in this setting, the patient was on the stage. He looked to be in his early sixties with straw-colored hair thinning on top. He wore a plain beige shirt with an open collar and pale khaki chinos. Except for the speaker at the podium, the man sat alone, looking bewildered and anxious, his eyes scanning the audience. He was not in a hospital gown, which told me he had been discharged from the hospital and must have been asked to come back to attend this conference.

The chief resident told us the man had emigrated from the Ukraine to São Paolo, Brazil, where he plied his trade as a cobbler for 15 years. Each day during that period, he took the same bus route to and from the inner city—accompanied by lepers who were being treated as outpatients in São Paolo's leprosarium. He eventually immigrated to Seattle, where he was employed in a downtown shoe-repair shop.

About a year after arriving in Seattle, he developed heart failure. Fluid filling his lungs compressed them, making breathing difficult and labored. Having no health insurance, he sought help from the county hospital, Harborview, a teaching affiliate of the University of Washington medical school. He arrived at Harborview gasping for air. After only three days of aggressive treatment with digitalis and water pills, he was discharged in much improved condition. This short hospitalization was before the reduced length-of-stay imposed by HMOs (health maintenance organizations) or reimbursement to hospitals based on DRGs (diagnostic related groups) rather than length-of-stay even existed. The patient was told to report for a follow-up evaluation in the residents' teaching clinic in two weeks. The chief resident continued his description of the case. At the follow-up visit, the patient had a bump in his right temple area that was scaly in the center and slightly reddened along the rim. The residents noted the bump was directly over the temporal nerve. The patient told the residents he had no feeling in the area.

Soon after the follow-up evaluation, the patient was seen in the dermatology clinic by a staff dermatologist fresh out of her residency—and, like many newly minted specialists, she did everything by the book. She performed a biopsy of what the patient described as an enlarging growth. Several days later, the dermatologist received the pathology report describing the biopsy results. In a state of utter shock and amazement, she read that the submitted tissue was teeming with mycobacterium leprae, the bacterium that causes leprosy.

The patient was promptly admitted to University Hospital as a teaching case, which was a euphemism for a patient with high teaching value but no health insurance. Why he was not readmitted to Harborview is a matter of conjecture but must have created some friction within the system. In fact, in his Grand Rounds presentation of the patient's history and physical examination, the chief resident implied, in a thinly veiled manner, that the diagnosis of leprosy had been "missed" at Harborview, even though the diagnosis had been made before the patient was admitted to University Hospital. Apparently, there was a spirit of competition between the Harborview and University Hospital, despite the fact both hospitals were staffed by the same faculty and house staff.

After the chief resident completed his presentation, it was time for the discussion by the faculty member. In this instance, however, the discussant was a visiting specialist in infectious diseases from Harvard University who happened to be at the University of Washington for a job interview. He had been hand-picked by the chief of the university's Section of Infectious Diseases to be his successor. The chief was being elevated to the position of chairman of the department of medicine. It was the prevailing wisdom that only someone from Harvard could fill his shoes and perpetuate the sterling reputation of the Section of Infectious Diseases.

After a very dry, textbook discussion of the major types of leprosy—which I strongly suspect he read straight from a textbook—the discussant's opinion was the patient had contracted leprosy from very prolonged close contact (15 years) with the lepers on the bus in Sao Paolo. Ordinarily, leprosy is not easily transmitted. He also pointed out that he was surprised the biopsy of the lesion on the man's temple was rich with organisms for what he considered the tuberculoid form of leprosy. Usually this form, involving a nerve, contains a very limited number of bacteria. He quipped that the patient "had not read the book" (which I suspect he was reading from).

Then, the discussant from Harvard said to the audience, "If there are no questions, I invite any of you who have the guts to come up on the stage to touch and feel this guy. Don't worry, he doesn't understand or speak English."

There was stunned silence when, in a few rows in front of me, someone yelled, "Question in the back." Sitting next to the individual who yelled this, a gentleman with gnarled, arthritic hands and a stooped posture looked to be in his eighties. In retrospect (now knowing his identity), I estimate he was actually 65 at the time.

The man slowly struggled to stand by grasping the back of the seat in front of him. In a weakened voice, he began to make a comment when the discussant at the podium bellowed, "I can't hear a word he is saying. Will someone shove a microphone in front of him?" The person sitting at the end of the row unhooked a microphone from a stand in the aisle, and the microphone, wires and all, was tediously passed-in about eight seats.
The gentleman standing spoke into the mike. "Doctor, that was certainly a very complete description of the different types of

leprosy. I do have one minor point of disagreement. You have classified the patient as having the earlier tuberculoid stage of leprosy. I agree that the lesion on his temporal nerve is consistent with tuberculoid leprosy, as you have pointed out. I, too, would not expect it to be loaded with (M. leprae) organisms if this was, indeed, the tuberculoid form. However, his face is shiny and full. There are ridges and furrows on his forehead, and his cheeks are swollen. This leonine (lion-like) face is typical of the more advanced and more infectious lepromatous form of leprosy in which we would expect the abundance of mycobacterium."

Instead of a "thank you for that clarification, doctor", the discussant said in an arrogant and patronizing tone, "And how do you come by that knowledge, doctor?"

By this time, the gentleman making the comment was already seated. Once again, as he slowly rose to his feet, the microphone was brought to him. He said, "I am Dr. Norman Sloan. I was the medical director of the Kalaupapa Leprosarium on the island of Molokai for 20 years." He then plopped back into his seat.

Although retired, Dr. Sloan was undoubtedly at the University of Washington meeting for the continuing medical education and intellectual stimulation offered by the Grand Rounds. Few physicians are able to abandon their identity and persona as a doctor in his retirement years.

After Dr. Sloan spoke, everyone in the amphitheater rose to their feet for a standing ovation. People gathered around him, plying him with questions for over an hour. The pretender to the throne from Harvard put his tail between his legs and exited stage left, never to be seen again. His head rolled that day—he was not offered the position of chief of infectious diseases.

A final thought: Arrogance diminishes wisdom—Arabian proverb.

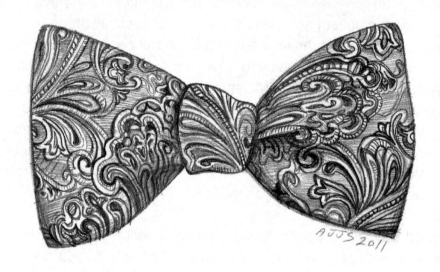

Bow Ties

A shoebox found on a shelf, filled with 20 mint-condition bow ties my late father had worn—little did I know what an impact they would have on me for the rest of my life. My father died of stomach cancer in 1957 at the age of 55, two and a half months before my 19th birthday. I was two weeks into my sophomore year of college. Thirty years later, at the age of 76, my mother suffered a frontal lobe brain hemorrhage which rendered her no longer able to live independently. She had lived in her home in Yonkers, New York, for 35 years.

Thanks to a letter from her kind and understanding attending physician at Bronxville Hospital, I transported her by air directly from the hospital to my home in Bloomfield Hills, Michigan. The letter assured the airline she was fit to travel by air and she would be accompanied by her son, a physician. It freed the airline from any responsibility if an untoward event should occur in flight. Furthermore, it guaranteed her a seat on the aisle in the first row behind the bulkhead, which had more room, and she could be literally carried with a special chair the short distance from the seat to a waiting wheelchair in the jetway. I made sure she went to the restroom before leaving the hospital and was wearing Depends in preparation for the one hour flight. Fortunately, there were no delays. My wife was able to assist us in that regard upon our arrival in Detroit.

As my mother's power of attorney and first-born son, one of my responsibilities was to sell her home in Yonkers and move her belongings to my home. We had already built a "handicap equipped" addition to our home two years prior to entice her to live with us but it remained unused. Now she could no longer resist losing her independence since the hemorrhagic stroke made the decision for her.

Clearly, the most difficult task I faced was removing the contents of my sister's room. She was killed in an automobile accident in March 1965 while commuting from college during her senior year. Carole planned to be a teacher with a degree in elementary education. In her closet, in addition to her mementos and personal belongings, a shoebox sat on the shelf. In it were 20 mint-condition bow ties that had been worn by my father. My mother had saved them for 30 years. I separated that shoebox from the rest of the contents of the home that were to be put in the moving van and placed it my car along with other precious memorabilia for the 900 mile drive back to Michigan. It was put on a shelf in my dressing closet where, although I acknowledged its presence daily, it remained unopened for almost a year until I had a last-minute need for a bow tie for a black tie event. Verifying there was a formal black bow tie in the shoe box, I went to Whaling's, exclusive men's clothier in Birmingham, to ask directions for tying a bow tie. They promptly produced instructions and were so helpful I felt obligated to purchase a bow tie from them.

Frankly, I had considerable difficulty in tying the very shiny, smooth and slippery black bow tie. I subsequently learned this texture is definitely not the ideal trainer bow tie. Ultimately, my struggle was successful and the bow saved the day, or should I say, night.

From that point on, I wore one of my father's bow ties with a frequency only often enough to maintain my skills in tying one. About a year later, I attended a medical seminar where Dr. John Canine, a psychotherapist, was addressing the topic of normal and abnormal grieving in response to the loss of a loved one. He was a gifted speaker whose practice was limited to grief counseling. Many of his patients were referred by funeral homes as well as bereaved families concerned about one of their members. He brought up the concept of linking objects.

In 1972, psychoanalyst Vamik Volkan had coined the term "linking object" to describe what is usually an inanimate object that connects a mourner, in a comforting way, to a deceased loved one. Naturally, caring for a pet of the deceased would serve as a live linking object. It can serve to maintain a healthy bond of remembrance that can have intimate meaning only to the mourner. The article is either carried on the person or worn by the bereaved individual or placed on a bureau or mantle where it is seen with regularity. Examples for men would be something that the deceased used regularly such as a watch, medal or key chain or an article of clothing. For women it might be a piece of jewelry such as a bracelet, necklace or ring. For either sex, it might be a photo, letter or gift they had received from the deceased. It is whatever has meaning to you and is symbolically linked to your lost loved one so they are never out of your mind and heart. It is a tool to bring empathy, understanding and awareness that love never dies. It may represent a common bond or extension of your personality to your lost loved one. It can be an active continuing link that provides continuing access to a defining personality characteristic of your deceased mother or father. It may be representative of one of their characteristics that you identify in yourself. For many, it can be a transitional tool to assist the mourner having difficulty coping with the separation until it is no longer needed.

Although most linking objects are selected soon after one's loss, mine was identified almost 30 years after my father's death at the age of 50. It was not until I was made aware of the utility of linking objects in maintaining an active continuous link to my father. Despite the bow tie being a positive linking object to my father, for almost a half century, I had been unable to view any linking objects to my sister such as her photo or charm bracelet without sadness, tears and some anger. She died in an automobile accident at the age of 22. My release came when I gifted my sister's charm bracelet to my first granddaughter, Caroline Grace, on the day of her baptism. It was as if Carole Ann was symbolically reborn. Volkan has pointed out that linking objects can also hinder or delay satisfactory resolution of the grieving process. They are not always useful or positive and can open psychological wounds but not heal them. Grieving is such a highly individualized and personalized process.

Wearing a bow tie has now become part of my persona and the image I wish to project. I wore one every day in my professional capacity ever since learning about its significance as a linking object. In my retirement, the practice continues. Out of respect for my doctors and the medical profession, I wear a sport coat and bow tie to every office visit and whenever I visit someone in the hospital. For Sunday Mass, weddings, funerals, baptisms, confirmations and the Friday meetings of the Senior Men's Club of Birmingham, I wear a bow tie with a suit or sport coat. My collection now numbers 365, theoretically one for each day of the year but many are used repeatedly because they are my favorites or go so well with what I wear regularly. To avoid being accused of having a fetish instead of being a collector, if I purchase another bow tie from a store, catalog or the Internet that I must have, I give one away (with instructions) to those I think would look good in a bow or who have shown interest in joining the elite ranks of bow tie wearers.

Bow ties reached their peak of popularity in the 1930s. Long ties— also known as four-in-hand ties—and bow ties were fairly equal in popularity. In the '40s and '50s, Frank Sinatra maintained the popularity of bows for those hoping to achieve his popularity with the bobbysoxers. In the '60s, bow ties degenerated into the pop-art and Op-art craze. They received bad press in the '70s and '80s unless being worn with formal clothes. At that time, John T Molloy, syndicated fashion columnist, lecturer and author of Dress for Success warned, "If you wear a bow tie you will not be taken seriously when wearing one. Most people will not trust you with anything important." Even worse he gratuitously added, "In general, I have found that people believe that a man in a bow tie will steal." He went on to write that bow tie wearers are seen as outsiders, self-styled mavericks, intellectuals and pompous academics who "lack credibility and validity as speakers—men who will never rise to the pinnacle of corporate power." Molloy wrote, "You may as well wear a red nose and a beanie as wear a bow tie. The number of people who will trust you at all, with anything, will automatically be cut in half." This was almost a lethal blow to the bow tie wearer since Time magazine called Molloy "America's first wardrobe engineer."

Fifteen years ago, John Spooner wrote in the Atlantic monthly, "I know that bow tie people tend to be short men who appear to be cock-sure of themselves." Bow tie wearers were thought to be less virile than the long-tie wearer by conservative straight-arrow types who believe those who sport a bow tie have a tendency toward irresponsibility and are scatterbrains. The bow tie became associated with mad professors and noisy advertising men whom few wanted to imitate.

Though the bow tie has been around longer than the dominant four-in-hand tie, it has existed for years on the brink of extinction—an endangered butterfly (pun intended). It was kept alive by a cult of devotees representing a tiny percentage of the necktie wearing public. In 1993, 3-5 percent of the 200 million ties sold in this country were bow ties. In 2005, that figure dropped to only 2 percent. The number of men wearing long ties has dropped even more dramatically with the advent of business casual in the workplace. Bow ties had already lost favor in the business community because they are complicated to tie and cannot be loosened. Also, the tendency to conformity has guided most men's choices for business attire. The bow tie is not synonymous with conformity. Corporate commanders demand conformity and compliance from their employees and the bow tie is seen as a threat. Corporations don't want a non-conformist in their ranks—someone who is not a team player. The stereotype is that he might be extremely bright and exactly what the corporation needs but is feared because of his individualistic behavior which might have a disruptive influence on the organization. He might not go along with its traditional policies and practices. Others may follow and that is frightening because the corporation fears loss of control. For these reasons, the bow tie has been thought to be a corporate no-no.

Admittedly, bow ties are not for everyone. They are controversial. It takes confidence, courage, craftsmanship, charm and, perhaps, a bit of cunning to master tying a bow. It should never be worn by a man who is self-conscious. Bow tie wearers enjoy swimming against the tide. Five years ago, Bill Kennerson, founder of Beau Ties Ltd of Burlington, Vermont, told me the following about the demographics of his ties. "A person who wears a bow tie is someone who wants to be noticed, who is different, who wants to stand out, who has an independent streak, who is not self conscious" In 2005, he sold 60,000 bow ties. Of these 26 percent were sold in New England; 14 percent in New York, Pennsylvania and Delaware; 13 percent in D.C., Maryland, Virginia and the Carolinas and 12 percent in the Northwest and California.

Bill Blass, the fashion authority, said bow tie wearers are, "A cult, a signature look for intellectuals, a highly personal signature." Washington lawyer, Mark Sandground, who wears bow ties himself, says bow ties aren't the thing to look for in a juror. "If they wear a frown, that's when you are in trouble." I guess that wearing this particular piece of wearing apparel bespeaks a very expressive body language.
In 2007 and 2008, Russell Smith, style columnist for the Toronto Globe and Mail, said, "Left-wingers recoil at what they perceive to be a symbol of political conservatism." He argues the anachronism

is the point and bow tie wearers are making a public statement that they disdain changing fashion. In Smith's view, the bow tie is "the embodiment of propriety and an indicator of fastidiousness and intelligence."

Obviously, a stereotype persists that intellectual, even nerdy, types gravitate toward bow ties since they are especially favored by intellectuals and creative professionals. In his book, *Proof of Heaven*, Eben Alexander, MD, offers this perception of a bow tie wearer. Shortly after his near-death experience from bacterial meningitis (inflammation of the covering of the brain and spinal cord), he was evaluated by a neurologist for rehab placement. Dr. Alexander, a neurosurgeon, wrote that the neurologist "insisted that I was 'too euphoric' and that I was probably suffering from brain damage. This doctor, like me, was a regular bow-tie wearer, and I returned the favor of his diagnosis by telling my sisters, after he had left, that he was 'strangely flat of affect for a bow-tie aficionado'."

"But the person who wears a bow is often independent, well educated, in a position of power and confidant enough to express his individuality" says Kirk Hinckley, president of the Bow Tie Club. From his August 26, 2011 newsletter, *The Bow Tie Times*, the following is reprinted with his permission.

"Ode to the Bow Tie

This Sunday August 28th is a very special day, it is National Bow Tie Day and it put me to thinking why I started wearing bow ties and what makes them so special! One main reason is the connection a bow tie affords people and what I mean by that is the bow tie wearers giving of themselves to the viewer, we open up a door to our lives when we wear a bow tie, we are exposing a small part of who we are in the world. You see a bow tie wearer and you see an individualist, a person who has the freedom to express themselves at their job, you see a person who is not afraid to break from the mold of traditional men's fashion.

I believe this sharing is what makes a bow tie wearer a little more approachable than most. The information that a bow tie conveys helps start that conversation with a stranger, it creates the smile on the child and it becomes a catalyst to remember the meeting of someone new. If you wear a bow tie to a job interview, the bow tie helps attach the person to their skills. A salesperson in a bow tie will be remembered by the customer and the bow tying politician will always stand out from the crowd!

So I thank you bow tie for all the women who could not help but straighten you over the years. All the conversations you have helped start with complete strangers and for not dipping into my soup at lunchtime like so many long ties did in my pre-bow years!

But most importantly, I thank you for the smile you bring to my daughter's face when she sees daddy wearing a new bow tie!

So my fellow bow tiers, I ask you to take a moment this Sunday to reflect on what the bow tie has done for you, the smiles, the memories and the people you have met while donning this intriguing and beautiful symbol of who we are!"

Traditionally, bow ties are associated with certain professions such as architects, attorneys, university professors, teachers and politicians. They are also favored by physicians, especially pediatricians. Pediatricians feel more approachable and children friendly but, importantly, kids can't grab their ties and infants can't pee on them. Surgeons choose them to avoid dragging germs on a long tie from patient to patient, especially during minor surgery and wound dressings. Bow ties are a favorite of pathologists and hematologists who spend hours looking into a microscope. An article in the July 13, 2012 Chicago Daily Law Bulletin by staff writer Pat Milhizer quotes Gregory L. Shugar, an attorney who runs TheTieBar.com as saying, "It just continues to pick up month over month. Our bow tie sales continue to grow." In fact, Chicago has a

Bow Tie Society which meets once a year at the Union League Club.

There are different sizes and styles of bow ties. It is important to pair the tie to the size of the neck and one's stature to create a proportionately balanced look. Personality is projected in style as much as it is in colors and patterns. The large butterfly bow (wing size 3-3.5 inches) is for the man with a large neck size and bigger face or chin. Please leave the large butterflies to the big and tall men. They are to be avoided if you don't meet that description unless you want to create a comic look, especially with bright colors and a wild pattern. Add large red polka dots and you will look like a clown. The classic or standard bow (wing size 2.25-2.75 inches) is a safe choice especially for black tie functions regardless of the wearer's height and weight. It is the most popular style. Narrow or slim-line bow ties also called "bat wings" (wing size 1.5-2.0 inches) look best on thin men with an elongated face and narrow collar size. Bow ties may have pointed ends (diamond point) and are acceptable for black tie events but have limited versatility. They tend to look old fashioned but some desire that look. The pointed ends are designed to stick out beyond the straight edge of the loops, requiring more finesse in tying them.

The length of a bow tie is adjustable with either buttons, as found on a Carrott and Gibbs bow, or hooks with eyelets marked with your neck size, as with Beau Ties Ltd bows. However, those of you with a neck size of 17 or above should notify the manufacturer in order to get a suitable length. The width or the distance between the two tips of a bow tie should be the same as that between the outer edges of your eyes and never be broader than the widest part of your neck. It should never extend past the tip of the shirt collar.

A pre-tied or ready-tied bow tie is either a bow sewn on to an adjustable band which goes around the neck or to a clip which attaches to the collar in front. One that is tied by hand is called freestyle, self-tie or tie-yourself. Alan Flusser, men's clothing designer and author of *Dressing the Man,* is quoted as saying, "Place a pre-tied model under your chin and you forsake any claim to individuality or style. It's like allowing someone to forge your signature." Clip-ons are a cop out, a con-man's dodge and are intellectually dishonest. The exceptions to these axioms are those crippled with arthritis or shaking with palsy who are well intentioned and whose heart is still with a bow tie. To say "I was a boy scout washout in knot-tying so I have to wear a clip-on" is unacceptable, as is "I find it more difficult than tying my shoelaces in the dark when I am drunk so I have to wear a pre-tied." A clip-on may be suitable for a 5-year-old who is being forced to have his picture taken by the mall photographer to send to grandma, but not beyond.

The same rules regarding color and pattern hold for bow ties as they do for standard neckties. The point in the business world is tasteful understatement. But sometimes they are meant to make a statement such as the stars and stripes on Independence Day and certain national holidays. Personally, I have 12 bow ties with a Christmas theme for each of the 12 days of Christmas, one for Halloween, Thanksgiving and Valentine's Day, and a stars and stripes bow tie. There are bows designed as gifts from well-intentioned clients and patients for attorneys, architects, physicians and pharmacists.

When bow tie enthusiasts talk about this piece of cloth around their neck, they speak with the dedication of those who have found religion. To them it is more of a fashion than a fad. The bow tie battalion is built on a tradition of not being trendy. Admittedly, retailers say most bow tie wearers are over the age of 40. Perhaps it takes a certain number of years for the seasoning process to give us the courage to stand out and develop an independent sense of ourselves. More recently, many college age students are starting to wear them but they are making it the centerpiece of their outfit rather than an accessory that is color and pattern coordinated with their ensemble as a finishing touch. Sadly, some are too large for the stature of the wearer or look cartoonish. It is designed to stand out. Some of the faces donning a bow tie are even younger, such as Justin Bieber at the 2011 Grammy Awards.

Bow ties are definitely making a comeback. Randall Hanauer Jr. A manager along with his Dad, Randy, at R. Hanauer—a tie and pocket square company—says the 25-year-old firm saw its best year in 2010 and the figures are not yet in for 2011. The 2011 Golden Globes saw Robert DeNiro and Brad Pitt sporting bow ties. In response to business casual that has crept into the workplace, the bow tie is now re-emerging in that setting along with a sport-coat or suit. Since today's businessman can now want to dress, not need to, dressing outside the box could mean a color coordinated bow tie and pocket square.

A bow tie is like life itself. You have to play with it, tweak it to get it right. Even then, it's always a bit askew but it should be. You decide where you want to be in the bow tie spectrum. Are you a little polka dot guy who wears stripes on the weekend or are you a solid with figures of animals, golf clubs, scales of justice or caduceus. Perhaps a take-charge regimental stripe or Scottish plaid? In any event, a bow tie guy knows this and does not ask "what is the latest fashion or trend?" A bow tie reflects your personality, mood, temperament and self-image more than any other fashion accessory. Wear it with distinction.

A final thought: August 28 is National Bow Tie Day. It is also the feast of my patron saint, Augustine. I was named after my father!

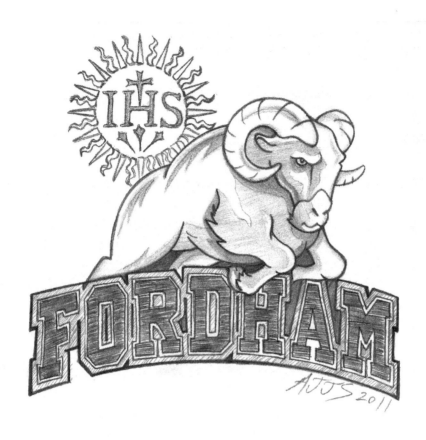

The Interview

The small thin man in the white suit and black tie sitting next to me on the Boeing 707 appeared to be quite anxious as we rolled down the runway at Idlewild (now JF Kennedy International) Airport on Long Island, New York, in November 1960. With a heavy Puerto Rican accent, he told me he was attending his brother's funeral in Chicago. I offered my condolences. In a naïve attempt to put him at ease, I told him this was my first airplane flight and I was naturally a bit fearful. My comments did not seem to diminish what was now a look of sheer terror on his face as we felt the plane leave the ground. He spent the rest of the flight reciting his rosary in Spanish and periodically making the sign of the cross. I indicated to him I was aware he was praying for his deceased brother's soul. He looked at me quizzically before replying he was praying for his own soul because this was also his first airplane flight. Thankfully, the flight turned out to be rather uneventful.

I was on my way to an interview for admission to the Chicago College of Osteopathy (CCO)—now Midwestern University/Chicago College of Osteopathic Medicine.

In those days, an airline ticket agent could also function as your travel agent and provide information about ground transportation, hotel options and even local restaurants. My agent and I determined that—based on my financial means (which were almost nonexistent)—the closest hotel to CCO I could afford was almost a mile from CCO's Basic Science Building, where I was to report the next morning at 8 a.m. Although it was sunny and pleasant when my plane landed at O'Hare Airport in Chicago, it snowed overnight—and it continued to snow as I made the long walk to the interview site. It was also very cold and windy, and I regretted not taking a hat with me.

Upon my arrival at the Basic Science Building, I was greeted by the registrar, Mrs. Virginia Costello. As she offered to take my snow-covered coat and scanned me up and down, she must have noticed my well-shined-shoes had just endured a grueling trek through the snow. I was apparently the last of the interviewees to arrive. The other seven students, sitting quietly in the office, seemed to be fresh and alert, as if they had not battled the elements as I had. They must have driven to the site, I thought.

For some reason, Mrs. Costello continued the conversation with me. Fortunately, I addressed her as Mrs. Costello and not by her first name. I was unaware at the time that my social skills, poise and comportment were being critically assessed by her, and her input was highly valued by the admissions committee. The biblical admonition, "The first shall be last and the last shall be first," came to mind when she directed me to start the interview process in an adjoining lounge. Little did I know what was in store for me there.

70

Upon entering the lounge, I noticed two interviewers, both young men. One greeted me with a handshake and introduced himself as Dr. Melvin Fritz. With a Brooklyn accent, he introduced me to Dr. Terence Sullivan, who was sitting in a chair by the wall. He smiled and nodded a silent gesture of greeting. Dr. Fritz suggested I take a seat on the large couch while he sat behind a desk.

Before I could feel the cushion of the couch under my derriere, Dr. Fritz blurted out, "Jesuit high school, Jesuit college…you're not going to find any of that Jesuit stuff around here."

I said, "I beg your pardon?"

He responded by asking, "Don't you think that your religion would pose a handicap in the practice of medicine?"

I replied, "My code of medical ethics may come in conflict with requests from some of my patients, but by following the dictates of my conscience, I would not be prevented from practicing according to ethical guidelines."

"Ah ha," he said, "you admit that your sense of what is morally right might conflict with your patient's. In what areas do you think there may be a conflict?"

At this point, I came to two conclusions: First, I was not going to be accepted into this school, and second, Dr. Fritz equated ethics with morality, and he believed morals are based on religious beliefs.

I really wanted to be accepted to this school but felt thoroughly intimidated. Yet, thinking I now had nothing to lose, I went after Dr. Fritz with both barrels.

I answered his question by noting that medical ethics defines a code of conduct the medical profession adheres to. It is a body of principles the profession uses to decide which behaviors are right, good and proper. An ethical principle does not always dictate a single course of action. Moral values can come into conflict with actions deemed medically ethical. The classic example today would be abortion. Abortion is now legal (though it was not at the time of my interview). Therefore, abortion is deemed to be medically ethical, but a physician may find it personally immoral.

To some people, morals are subjective judgments based on one's religious, cultural and philosophical concepts and beliefs. However, I believe morals are a system of standards used to produce honest, decent and ethical results based on the theory of natural law. The theory of natural law aids us in understanding which human actions are morally right or wrong based on human reason alone—not on divine revelation, religious dogma, philosophical premises, human emotions or personal opinions. Natural law is not an attempt to impose one's ethical system on another person or profession. It is grounded in the fact that human nature allows us to know what is good or bad for us as individuals and as members of the community.

Natural law is the same for all of us, and its fundamental concepts cannot be changed, because our human nature cannot be changed. Natural law applies to people regardless of time, culture, background, race, sex, religion or political affiliation. However, an individual's morality and ethics must be consistent with his or her religious beliefs. Otherwise—in my case—I would be a shopping cart Catholic, picking off the shelf what I liked that was within easy reach and leaving what was not easy to reach.

Fortunately, I was armed in my interview with a course in medical ethics I had taken during my senior premedical year at Fordham College. The course was taught by Father Edward McNally, a Jesuit priest and a lawyer. Father McNally was the brother of the actor, Steve McNally, best remembered for his roles—usually as the villain and occasionally as the hero—in western and action movies of the 1940s and 1950s. Both brothers were graduates of

Fordham Law School. Steve practiced law for several years before pursuing his childhood dream of becoming an actor. Edward followed his boyhood dream and became a Jesuit priest.

Father McNally taught his classes in a peripatetic, Aristotelian style. The students' desks were arranged in a circle. He would walk around vigorously within the circle, facilitating the discussion by bringing up a subject and then pointing to an individual to respond to his provocative question. This was usually followed by pointing to another student to respond to the first student's comment.

Our class became a debate team that discussed logic, philosophy, morality and medical ethics, guided by the teachings of the Roman Catholic faith emanating from a razor-sharp mind. Father McNally never shrank from ambiguity, and he was able to confront moral dilemmas with the skill of a surgeon wielding Occam's razor. Occam's (or Ockham's) razor is a principle attributed to the 14th-century Franciscan friar, William of Ockham. The most useful explanation of this principle, often noted by scientists, is: when you have two competing theories that make exactly the same predictions, the simpler theory is the better one. In essence, select the option that makes the fewest assumptions.

My interview with Dr Fritz covered the spectrum of abortion, euthanasia, artificial insemination and birth control. But in 1960, medical abortion, the morning-after pill, physician-assisted suicide, fetal and embryonic stem-cell research, cloning, genetic engineering and sex selection were not in our vocabulary as issues to be reckoned with.

Dr. Fritz raised the ethical question of whether a physician can pursue a good effect while knowing it will or may cause a bad effect. He used the example of performing an abortion when a woman has an ectopic pregnancy. In most cases, an ectopic pregnancy is when a human embryo implants in one of the two fallopian tubes instead of in the lining of the uterus (womb). In considering this example, I invoked the principle of double effect.

73

Under this principle, I related that the following five conditions must be present simultaneously for a medical action to be morally acceptable:

1. The action, in itself, must be good, or at least not morally evil (i.e., it can be morally neutral or indifferent).

2. The good effect cannot be obtained in some alternate way without producing harm or evil.

3. The good effect must not be the result of an evil means or, to put it another way, the evil act cannot be the means for producing the good effect.

4. The evil effect is not willed, but merely permitted.

5. There must be a reasonably grave reason for permitting the evil effect—a proportionately grave reason for performing the action.

Up to 70 percent of ectopic pregnancies resolve spontaneously with the death of the embryo. However, ruptured ectopic pregnancies account for about 6 percent of all pregnancy related deaths. From a Catholic perspective, watchful waiting with close monitoring (i.e., expectant management) is an acceptable way of handling such pregnancies. No direct or intended killing of the embryo is involved, and there is no moral problem unless the mother's life is unnecessarily put at risk. If the ectopic pregnancy does not resolve spontaneously, then another means of resolving the problem is needed to protect the life of the woman.

One type of treatment for a woman with an ectopic pregnancy is removal of all or part of the fallopian tube with the embryo inside (a procedure known as salpingectomy). It is clear this procedure is morally acceptable by applying the principle of double effect. If the embryo continues to grow in the fallopian tube, rupture of the tube and possible death of the mother and unborn child may result.

When the tube or a portion of it is removed, the death of the embryo is unintended.

Another type of treatment is salpingostomy, the removal of an embryo from the fallopian tube while leaving the tube intact. This procedure is often considered for the woman whose other fallopian tube is blocked or absent—to preserve the woman's future fertility. Although this procedure is morally acceptable if the embryo has already died, it is not acceptable if the embryo is still alive, because it involves the direct killing of an innocent human being. The distinction between salpingostomy and salpingectomy is the distinction between intending the death of the living embryo and merely foreseeing that death as a result of the medical treatment.

The interview moved on to questions about my reading preferences and my taste in movies. I was also asked to explain my thesis on the biochemical genetics of sickle cell anemia, which I wrote while taking graduate-level courses at New York University's Graduate School of Arts and Sciences. As I described my thesis in great depth to try to impress the doctors, I recall Dr. Fritz, with eyes glazed, saying, "It has been quite a while since Dr. Sullivan and I have thought about that subject."

My rather extensive interview with Dr. Fritz lasted about a half hour. During that entire time, Dr. Sullivan just sat there grinning and saying absolutely nothing—but it turned out he was surely listening.

When Dr. Fritz terminated the interview, Dr. Sullivan, once again, nodded and smiled without saying a word. I thought I had held my own during the interview and had answered all the provocative questions from Dr. Fritz with a clarity and conviction derived from my educational experience with Father McNally.

The remaining four interviews I had that morning were with individuals considerably older than doctors Fritz and Sullivan. They went well and really picked up my spirits, now thinking I had a chance to be accepted. After lunch, the other seven interviewees and I reported to a classroom, where we were administered the Minnesota Multiphasic Personality Inventory (MMPI). Our proctors were, once again, doctors Fritz and Sullivan. We were given up to an hour and a half to complete the test. This was followed by a tour of the Basic Science Building and the Chicago Osteopathic Hospital and Clinic.

The MMPI is frequently used by clinical psychologists and psychiatrists to assist in identifying personality structure and psychopathology. It is also used as a screening instrument for certain professions, including the osteopathic medical profession and high-risk occupations, such as first responders (e.g., police, firefighters, emergency medical technicians). The test should preferably be administered, scored, and interpreted by a psychologist or psychiatrist who has had specific training in the use of the MMPI.

Historically, the role and mission of colleges of osteopathic medicine (COMs) have been directed to the education of primary care physicians. For this reason, people skills are considered essential. The ability to relate to patients by using good communication skills is considered an important selection factor in the interview process for COMs. The MMPI can aid in evaluating this ability.

The 10 clinical scales as measured by the MMPI (which are numbered 1 to 0, rather than 1 to 10) are:

1. perception and preoccupation with one's health and health issues

2. level of depressive symptoms

3. awareness of one's problems and vulnerabilities

4. conflict, struggle and anger about, and respect for, society's rules
5. stereotypical masculine or feminine interests and behaviors
6. levels of trust, suspiciousness and sensitivity

7. levels of worry, anxiety, tension, doubts and obsessiveness

8. unusual or odd cognitive, perceptual and emotional experiences

9. level of excitability

0. whether one enjoys and is comfortable with being around other people

Despite my doubts during the interview with Dr. Fritz, I was accepted into CCO. Flash forward to 1964, when I was in my third year at CCO and taking a mixture of didactic classes and outpatient clinics. During our clinical rotations, my fellow students and I were assigned obstetric patients. We were expected to provide prenatal care to the patients under the supervision of an obstetrician/gynecologist (OB/GYN) and to be present during each patient's labor and delivery. Our patients with gynecologic problems were brought to the OB/GYN clinic, where we participated in their examination and implemented treatment recommendations under supervision.

On the first day of my rotation, I reported to the chief resident in OB/GYN for an orientation and tour of the obstetrics suite. I was directed to the OB/GYN lounge. As soon as I walked in, I recognized the chief resident as Dr. Terence Sullivan, the silent interviewer. Introducing myself, I mentioned he was one of my interviewers for admission to the college in November 1960. But I added, "Not really, because you never said a word during the entire interview." He didn't recall it at all. Then I said, "Dr. Melvin Fritz really did all the talking. You just sat there with a smile during the ordeal."

He asked me, "What did Fritz say?"

I replied, "Well, for openers, he said, 'Jesuit high school, Jesuit college…you're not going to find any of that Jesuit stuff around here.' "

"Oh, my God," Dr. Sullivan exclaimed, "you were the guy from Fordham!"

"Yes," I answered, "that's right. You do remember."

His eyes lit up and that broad Irish grin came back. He then told me, "You kicked the crap out of Fritz. I was so proud of you. Let me tell you what was going on.

"We weren't even doctors at the time. We didn't graduate until 1962. We were third-year students who had a research grant from the department of psychiatry. Our study objective was to determine whether we could predict a candidate's profile on the MMPI from our admission's interview with the candidate. The results were interpreted in a single-blinded manner by Dr. Elsa Johnson, the chairman of the psychiatry department." Single-blinded means the interpreter was unaware of the findings of the interviewers when she scored each candidate's responses.

Dr. Sullivan continued, "We decided that the person to interview the candidates was the one most unlike them in background, culture and religion. Mel interviewed you because I'm a graduate of Loyola High School and Loyola University—both Jesuit schools, as you know."

He then admitted, "Frankly, our research project was a disaster. We were all over the map in our predictions. I guess there is no substitute for a standardized and well-validated test. That wasn't us. Our evaluation of you didn't even count in the interview process."

Dr. Sullivan and I ended up developing a very productive professional relationship. And my clinical and hospital rotations in OB/GYN at CCO turned out to be among my best learning experiences—thanks to the personal attention of the "doctor" who was a silent interviewer in 1960.

A final thought: When the Bill of Rights was ratified, religious freedom had the distinction of being the First Amendment. We have a God-given, legally recognized right not to be forced to act in a manner contrary to our beliefs.

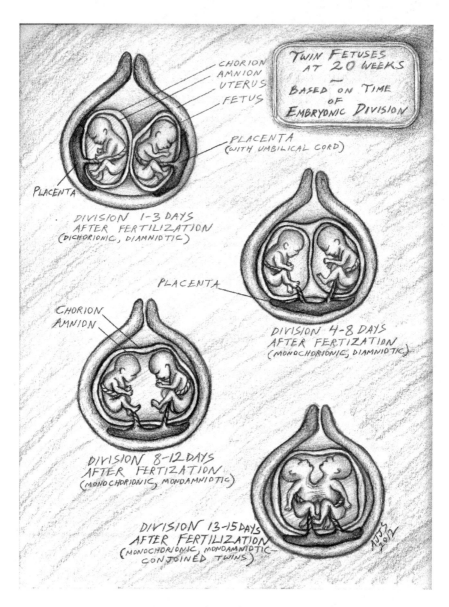

Labels in figure:

CHORION
AMNION
UTERUS
FETUS

TWIN FETUSES AT 20 WEEKS
BASED ON TIME OF EMBRYONIC DIVISION

PLACENTA (WITH UMBILICAL CORD)

PLACENTA

DIVISION 1-3 DAYS AFTER FERTILIZATION
(DICHORIONIC, DIAMNIOTIC)

PLACENTA

CHORION
AMNION

DIVISION 4-8 DAYS AFTER FERTIZATION
(MONOCHORIONIC, DIAMNIOTIC)

DIVISION 8-12 DAYS AFTER FERTIZATION
(MONOCHORIONIC, MONOAMNIOTIC)

DIVISION 13-15 DAYS AFTER FERTILIZATION
(MONOCHORIONIC, MONOAMNIOTIC—CONJOINED TWINS)

Wombmates—Myths and Realities

My daughter, Grace, and her husband, Patrick Byrnes, were blessed with the birth of fraternal twins (twins from different eggs) on May 27, 2007. The birth of the boys, named Michael Augustine and William John, piqued my curiosity about the phenomenon of twinning. Actually, I had been interested in this subject since my elementary school days, as a result of the seating arrangements at St. Frances of Rome parochial school in the Bronx, New York.

From first through eighth grade, I sat close to the Ryan identical twins, Paul and Joseph. At St Frances—because seating at the school was always by alphabetical order-and no one's last name began with a Q—my seat position gave me the opportunity to observe the twins six hours a day for eight years. It was obvious to me and everyone in our class that one of the twins was a better student than the other. In fact, the difference in their academic abilities was the only way we could tell the brothers apart, since they were physically identical and could not be distinguished by their appearance, speech pattern, tone of voice, or even gait.

During my high school years, the Dworkin fraternal twins were friends of mine. They also seemed to be close friends to one another, and they did everything together. The two brothers could easily be distinguished by physical appearance, but they had incredibly similar personalities and interests—though one was a bit of a daredevil (the shorter one) and the other was more reserved. The taller boy had a more prominent nose. Their mannerisms were almost identical.

Throughout my life, I have met or learned of many other pairs of twins—and I have been struck by both the similarities and differences between the individuals of each pair, whether identical or fraternal.

Heather is a petite 21-year-old sales associate in Diamonds and Doggies, a unique little shop near the beach in Lauderdale by the Sea, Florida. She sells puppies while her associates sell diamond jewelry in the same store. Heather told me she and her twin sister, Jessica, were born three months prematurely in one sac. No one has difficulty distinguishing the sisters, because Jessica has a large telangiectasia (pattern of dilated blood vessels near the skin surface that forms a type of birthmark) in the center of her forehead. Heather said Jessica is also an inch taller with a distinctly different personality. According to Heather, she herself is mild-mannered, almost shy and reticent, whereas Jessica is aggressive, dominant and far more outgoing.

There are other interesting comparisons between the twin sisters. Heather has a drooping eyelid on her left eye, but Jessica's right eye has a drooping lid—though the color of their irises is the same. Heather combs her hair to the left, while Jessica combs her hair to the right. Heather is right-handed, and her sister is left-handed. Both sisters have pierced ears on each side, but Heather's left ear has multiple piercings, whereas Jessica has multiple piercings in her right ear. Heather has a tattoo on her left ankle, and Jessica has one on her right ankle. They both have piercings in the middle of their tongues and a tattoo in the midline of the back of their neck.

Heather claims heel prints of her and Jessica taken at birth show the whorls to be mirror images of one another. Heather believes she and her sister are identical but mirror image twins.

Dominick and Cindy Schiano also describe their twins, Mike and Max, as mirror images from one sac. Their sons are now 26 years old and live together in Manhattan. Cindy relates that during her pregnancy, she selected the name Max for the one "who was always punching and kicking" in the womb, and Michael for the one who was more docile. After birth, Michael rolled gently in his sleep while his brother thrashed about. Dominick thought the "newborns looked exactly alike. I could only tell them apart when they moved or showed any animation."

The brothers' heel prints taken at birth were mirror images, according to their parents, and Mike's left foot is larger than his right foot, while the opposite is true of Max's feet. This difference coincides with Mike being left-handed and Max being right-handed. Cindy reports they had their own twin language and "would talk all night" with a speech that was unintelligible to others. Both boys had blond hair that darkened with age, though they came to part their hair on opposite sides. When Mike lost a left front tooth, Max's right front tooth fell out "within hours."

Early in their school years, both Schiano brothers had to get glasses to correct their distance vision. Mike hated science, and English was a challenge for Max. After they grew up, Max attended the Rochester Institute of Technology, where he majored in film technology. Currently, he writes television scripts and edits films. By contrast, Mike attended the Fashion Institute of Technology in Manhattan, where he studied fashion design. His specialty is shoes and handbags.

To the casual observer, the personalities of the identical mirror image twins Mike and Max differ perceptibly, as does their speech pattern. However, to their mother, "they are the same."

Harrison and Robert Visscher were born in Grand Rapids, Michigan, eighty-four years ago. They are identical but not mirror image twins.

When carrying the twins, their mother suffered from what was called, at that time, toxemia of pregnancy. Beginning in the third month of pregnancy her blood pressure became elevated. Her hands, feet and face began to swell due to retention of fluid and a large amount of protein appeared in her urine. Toxemia was thought to be due to toxic (poisonous) substances in the blood, which has been disproven. It is now called preeclampsia. If the condition is marked by a convulsion it is called eclampsia. Preeclampsia is usually observed after 20 weeks of pregnancy but can occur earlier if the mother has a multiple pregnancy or has other risk factors such as hyperthyroidism. A twin pregnancy almost triples the risk of preeclampsia and triplets triple the risk of preeclampsia compared with a twin pregnancy.

Harrison and Robert's mother, who wore the pants in the family, named Harry after the obstetrician who delivered the twins—Dr. Harrison Collisi. His brother was named, Robert Dale, after an attorney in the law office where she worked as his executive secretary. Their mother expected Harrison C. Visscher to be a doctor and Robert D. Visscher to be a lawyer.

From birth, the twins were raised to be identical in every way. Harrison said, "We slept in the same bed and were dressed in identical clothing until we got married at the age of 24." Their mother always maintained what Harrison describes as "a perfect balance and sense of equality between us." When one received an accolade or honor that the other did not, she would display some form of favoritism to the one who did not receive the award. She was egalitarian in an attempt to make them equal in all aspects of their lives. The brothers were, in fact, extremely well matched in athletic prowess. In high school, they both lettered in three sports— football, baseball and basketball. At 6'2" they were especially valued for their basketball skills. To this day, they maintain their athleticism by facing each on the tennis court twice a week.

Harrison and Robert have been very close all their lives and claim they can anticipate one another. Harry says, "We are the best of friends but we are also each other's major critic. We are equally competitive, which I feel has helped us to stay at the top of our game athletically, academically and professionally. Our last competition will be who delivers whose eulogy."

Harrison has decided to write Robert's eulogy while Robert is still alive. In the event he predeceases Robert, he has requested his daughter to deliver it at Robert's funeral so he can remain competitive even in the afterlife.

Harrison and Robert attended Hope College in Holland, Michigan. Perhaps to their mother's chagrin, they did not completely follow her expectations for their future occupations. They both decided to be physicians, graduating together from the University of Michigan's Medical School. Harrison admits, with characteristic humility, that his grades throughout their formal schooling were 2/100 of a point below Robert's. Between their junior and senior year at the U of M, Robert married four days before their 24th birthday and Harrison married six days after their birthday.

Following medical school, the brothers interned at different Michigan hospitals. Prior to their induction into the Armed Forces they each spent five months working in different family practice offices. Harrison joined the Army and Bob served in the Navy. When they returned from the service, they both completed a residency in exactly the same field—obstetrics and gynecology. Harrison served his residency at Northwestern University in Chicago. Robert's residency was at Balboa Naval Hospital in San Diego, California. Upon completion of their residencies, Harry said, "Our mother won out. We returned to Grand Rapids, where we practiced together, were affiliated with the same hospitals and where we started an obstetrics and gynecology residency training program." Both have written several articles which have been published in prestigious medical journals.

Harrison spent the last 15 years of his career as director of education for the American College of Obstetricians and Gynecologists. His current interest is the integration of faith and science. He lectures to college classes, various professional organizations, and different religious denominations in order to promote the public's understanding of the relationship between science and faith and have a more in-depth understanding of the science of evolution.

Robert founded the first in-vitro fertilization (IVF) laboratory in Western Michigan at Blodgett Memorial Medical Center Hospital in Grand Rapids. He later became executive director of the American Fertility Society (now the American Society of Reproductive Medicine). Currently, he is the president and an instructor for the

National Embryo Donation Academy. His efforts are aimed at educating professionals about issues surrounding the donation or receipt of embryos with hopes of achieving pregnancy and having a family. He has a special interest in the fate of the 600,000 frozen human embryos in the U.S. that are the result of the success of fertility treatments and assisted reproductive technology over the past 34 years. While most are retained for future children by their genetic parents, approximately 2-3 percent are in limbo with uncertain futures. The bioethics of their fate is a subject of considerable debate. The options are: keep them frozen, thaw and dispose, donate to research or my personal choice-donate them to other infertile couples hoping to have a baby.

Yet another interesting case of twins comes from the world of celebrities. Mary-Kate and Ashley, the famous Olsen twins, are now 26 years old. They began their acting careers at the age of nine months on the television series *Full House*, which was popular in the late 1980s and early 1990s. They looked so similar as children and young teenagers that the public assumed they were identical twins. The fact that one girl was left-handed and the other was right-handed supported the idea they were identical mirror-image twins. However, the Olson sisters are actually fraternal twins, with physical differences that became more easily discernible as they entered their late teenage years. There are also personality and emotional differences, which became obvious in 2004, when 18-year-old Mary-Kate checked into rehab suffering from anorexia nervosa.

How Twins Develop

The individual offspring of a single pregnancy that results in multiple births is called a multiple. Thus, the mother of twins, triplets, quadruplets, etc. is called a mother of multiples. The product of a single birth is called a singleton. A twin is one of two offspring produced in the same pregnancy. Twins can be dizygotic (fraternal), developing when two eggs are independently fertilized by two sperm cells to form two zygotes, or monozygotic (identical), developing when a single embryo splits during cell division to form two embryos.

Fraternal Twins

During each of the monthly menstrual cycles of a woman in her child-bearing years, typically only one egg is released from either her right or left ovary in the process of ovulation. Occasionally, however, both ovaries will release an egg in the same month. If both eggs are fertilized, the result is fraternal twins. Because fraternal twins develop from two separate eggs fertilized by two different sperm cells, they each have their own placenta. They each grow inside a separate sac, which has two layers of membrane covering the developing baby—the amnion (inner membrane containing the amniotic fluid in which the fetus floats) and the chorion (outer membrane that becomes part of the placenta). Such twins are referred to as being diamnionic (meaning there are two amnions) and dichorionic (meaning there are two chorions). However, the identification of fraternal twins by detecting two placentas is reliable only in the early stages of pregnancy, because the separate placentas sometimes fuse later in pregnancy. Approximately two-thirds of spontaneously (without the use of assisted reproductive technology) conceived twins are fraternal twins.

There are three gender variations of fraternal twinning. Male-and-female twins form the most common variation. Female-and-female twins (sororal twins) make up the next most common variation of fraternal twins, and male-and-male twins are the least common fraternal twin variation. Female fraternal twins are more common than male fraternal twins despite the fact that in the U.S. 105 males are born for every 100 females. Females have a survival advantage over males at every age thereafter. In the year 2012, women outlived men by six years.

Fraternal twins may resemble each other physically, or they may look very different from each other—as would be the case with any other pairs of brothers or sisters from the same parents. They are

87

simply siblings who happen to be the same age. Fraternal twins share 50 percent of their genes. If raised together, they also share most aspects of their environment, including parenting style, education, culture, community and socioeconomic status. These environmental similarities may result in certain common personality traits between fraternal twins despite their genetic diversity.

If a woman has a family history of fraternal twins on either her mother's or father's side of the family, she may inherit a tendency to hyperovulate—that is, to release more than one egg from her ovaries during each monthly menstrual cycle. The women of the Yoruba ethnic group in Nigeria were thought to have the highest rate of fraternal twinning in the world, reportedly with 40 to 50 per thousand births. This figure turns out to be grossly exaggerated. A pair of scientists from England and the Netherlands created a twin database for 76 developing countries as of 2010. Since identical twinning occurs at a relatively constant rate of 3.5 to 4 per thousand across all human populations, the variations observed between countries is almost completely due to the variation in the rate of fraternal twinning. The western central African nation of Benin is now the world's twinning champion at 27.9 per thousand. Togo is number 2 at 21.4 per thousand and Nigeria came in third at 19 per thousand. The Dutch author of the study stated, "The especially high twinning seen in Benin might be linked to the Yoruba ethnic group which can be found in Benin as well as in Togo and Nigeria." The high rate of fraternal twinning in the Yoruba has been attributed to a genetic tendency to hyperovulate coupled with consumption of a specific species of indigenous yam (genus dioscorea) containing a phytoestrogen (plant estrogen), diosgenin, thought to stimulate the ovaries to release more than one egg each month. It is a misconception that this yam contains any actual hormone. Our adrenal glands synthesize a hormone called dihydroepiandrosterone (DHEA) our body uses to create the male hormones (androgens) and female hormones (estrogens). Although diosgenin is structurally similar to DHEA, which can be converted in the laboratory to hormones, it cannot be converted to hormones in our body and does not appear to have any effect on a person's hormone levels. If this yam connection was true, one wonders if ingestion of large amounts of soy and soy byproducts, which are also rich in phytoestrogens, might contribute to fraternal twinning. This has not been investigated.

In comparison, twinning is very low in Asia and Latin America with rates less than 8 per 1,000 births. The major exceptions are the Caribbean Islands, where there are many people of West African descent. Haiti had a rate of 14.1 per thousand births. In the United States, by contrast, only three pairs of fraternal twins occur per 1,000 deliveries resulting from spontaneous conception.

Obese women and tall women are more likely to have fraternal twins than are underweight women and short women. The chance of giving birth to fraternal twins increases with age, beginning at age 30 until age 38, when it decreases. Fewer than 2 percent of births to teenaged mothers are fraternal twins, compared to more than 20 percent of births to women aged 45 and older. The higher rates of fraternal twinning in older women may be related to the rise in follicle stimulating hormone levels that normally occurs with age. This hormone stimulates the growth of eggs in the ovary. The increase in twin births observed with increasing age may be related to the number of pregnancies experienced by the mother before the twin pregnancy. In the 4th or 5th pregnancy, the chances are higher than in the first or second pregnancy.

High rates of fraternal twinning may also be related to the fact older women are more likely to use assisted reproductive technology (ART) than younger women. Assisted reproductive technology includes the use of fertility-enhancing drugs, which stimulate the ovaries to release an increased number of eggs (ovulation induction) which enhance the chances of more than one fertilized egg implanting in the endometrium (lining of the uterus). Assisted reproductive technology also includes in vitro fertilization (IVF), in which multiple eggs are fertilized in the laboratory and then surgically implanted into a woman's uterus and intrauterine insemination.

With the advent of ART to help women become pregnant, the rate of fraternal twinning has increased dramatically in the United States. Published in the December 5, 2013, issue of the New England Journal of Medicine, the trends in and the magnitude of the contribution of fertility treatments before they were available from 1962 through 1966, publicly available data on births from 1971 through 2011, and data on in-vitro fertilization (IVF) from 1997 through 2011 were used to estimate the annual proportion of twins that were attributable to IVF and to non-IVF fertility treatments (ovulation induction and ovarian stimulation). From 1998 to 2011 the estimated proportion of twin births that were attributable to IVF increased from 10 percent to 17 percent (a 70 percent increase). The estimated proportion of twin births attributable to non-IVF fertility treatments increased from 16 percent in 1998 to 19 percent in 2011. Thus, in 2011, 36 percent of twin births resulted from conception assisted by fertility treatments. After adjusting for maternal age, the number of twin births had increased by a factor of 1.6 from 1971 to 2009.

As mentioned, only three pairs of fraternal twins per 1,000 deliveries occur as a result of spontaneous conception in the United States. With IVF, by contrast, there are about 21 pairs of fraternal twins for every 1,000 deliveries. It is estimated the number of children born after IVF now exceeds 5 million.

Sororal Sisters

Maria and Elena are sororal fraternal twins who were born to Kathy and George when their son, Jason, was 23 years old. The couple had been trying to conceive another child naturally for years, but to no avail. Diagnoses of secondary infertility, diminished ovarian reserve, and advanced maternal age were rendered.

After much soul-searching and counseling from physicians, clergy and a pastoral medical ethicist from the Archdiocese of Detroit, Kathy and George made several unsuccessful attempts at using intrauterine insemination, a procedure in which sperm are placed directly into the uterine cavity. It can be used to treat infertility as long as one fallopian tube is open to allow access of the sperm to the egg. When this procedure did not work for them, the couple tried IVF. After two failed attempts at IVF, the third try ended with a spontaneous abortion (a miscarriage). The fourth IVF attempt was successful, with two of six embryos being successfully implanted a week before Kathy's forty-third birthday.

The couple had no need for the form of ART known as intracytoplasmic sperm injection, nor did they request preimplantation genetic screening (PGS), or preimplantation genetic diagnosis (PGD). Intracytoplasmic sperm injection is a technique in which a single sperm is injected directly into the cytoplasm of a mature egg. This procedure is sometimes performed for couples in which the man has a low sperm count or couples who have had no success with conventional IVF. In PGS, a single cell is removed from an embryo three days after fertilization for genetic analysis, to determine if there are abnormalities in the number or structure of chromosomes. In PGD, one or more cells are removed from a preimplantation embryo to determine whether the embryo has a genetic mutation or other genetic abnormality inherited from one or both parents.

Both PGS and PGD are controversial procedures with moral and ethical implications. In the March 2012 issue of the American Journal of Bioethics, two bioethicists contend that parents undergoing IVF, who are carriers of severely disabling genetic disorders, are morally obliged to sift through their embryos to find one that does not have the disease. They state, "Prospective parents who make an independent decision to reproduce using IVF and who know or reasonably should know they are at substantial risk for transmitting a serious genetic anomaly to their offspring, may be subject to legal liability for failing to utilize PGD to avoid birthing a child who suffers grave harm from the hereditable condition." These bioethicists impose "a duty on IVF-reproducing parents to maximize the well-being of their future offspring by all reasonable means." They further declare that, "Shifting benefit outlays for significant post-birth health care to a far less costly preconception procedure strikes us a worthy public policy trade-off." I would interpret these statements to be in support of government mandated health insurance to cover PGS, PGD and the potential of obligatory termination of the pregnancy (abortion) if the genetic defect is found in either the egg, sperm or embryo. The prolife community has a conscientious objection to using public funds (tax revenues) under The Health Care Affordability Act (Obamacare) or Medicaid for medical or surgical abortions as well as the destruction of a human embryo. One of several commentaries by bioethicists on that article, published in the same issue, would extend PGS and PGD to all "at risk" sources of eggs, sperm and embryos as a moral obligation and public duty, not just IVF-reproducing parents. For those of us who would not choose abortion and who believe human life begins at conception, PGS and PGD are not only superfluous but are morally objectionable. In addition, the processes may result in the loss of some embryos because of technical problems, and genetic tests sometimes yield false negative or false positive results.

Kathy's pregnancy was fraught with multiple, potentially life-threatening complications. She experienced three episodes of significant bleeding, attributed to a complete placenta previa (the blocking of the cervix opening by the placenta), at 19, 21 and 23 weeks into her pregnancy. At least one of these episodes required hospitalization, when massive bleeding occurred at 35 weeks. As Kathy and George were en route to the hospital in the early morning hours, another vehicle, traveling at about 70 miles per hour, nearly broadsided their van. They were quite shaken by the experience but, fortunately, escaped injury. Because of the previously diagnosed placenta previa, an emergency Caesarean section was performed on Kathy at about 4 a.m. The bleeding was controlled with a figure-eight suture, thereby avoiding the need for a hysterectomy. No additional measures were required, nor were there any further complications. Mom was discharged in four days, and the twins were brought home in two weeks. They were breast-fed.

Maria and Elena are now healthy and beautiful 12-year-old young ladies. Maria is taller than Elena by two to three inches and has similar features to her brother, Jason, with brown hair and brown eyes. She has an outgoing personality and loves reading books. Elena is quiet and shy with light brown hair and blue-green eyes, like her maternal grandfather. She is excellent in spelling and advanced math, like her mother.

Both twins are academically all A's. They appear to have inherited the ability to play a musical instrument from their parents. The twins both play the clarinet. And they are both athletic. Maria played basketball with her church league and is now trying softball. Elena also played basketball and has good hand-eye coordination. Both girls have been involved with the Girl Scouts for the past six years. Maria and Elena share these similarities despite efforts of their parents to split them up in school and other activities. Their grandparents expect they will become doctors, like their mother.

These sororal sisters are now enrolled in the Michigan State University Twin Registry, in which researchers are examining developmental differences in twins as they relate to genetic, environmental and neurobiological influences. Information on this study is available at www.msutwinstudies.com1index.html.

Identical Twins

One-third of all twins are identical. Identical twins result from the union of one egg and one sperm, forming a single zygote that splits into two embryos. The conventional wisdom is that identical twins are 100 percent genetically identical individuals. Although identical twins share the same DNA—making them carbon copies of each other—it is well established that genetic differences do exist between identical twins. In some cases, identical twins may express different phenotypes, such as skin color or height, because of activation or deactivation of different genes in each twin during development. Identical twins always share the same sex, blood type, and hair color, unless genetic mutations occur during embryonic development.

In spontaneous pregnancies, the incidence of identical twins is fairly uniform throughout the world, at about 3 to 5 per 1,000 live births (0.3 to 0.5 percent). In the U.S., the incidence is one in 240 (0.41 percent) of naturally conceived births. The rate of identical twins conceived through IVF is six times higher—at about 2.3 percent.

While waiting in line at the post office in Birmingham, Michigan, I chatted with a mother and her triplets—two girls and a boy—who were about two years old. In the course of our conversation, the mother volunteered that the children had been conceived with IVF. The girls were obviously identical twins, and the boy was fraternal. This results when one of two implanted fertilized eggs splits to form identical twin girls, both of whom are fraternal to the other fertilized male embryo. The mother told me her obstetrician had informed her "there was about a one out of 5,000 chance" of this triplet combination occurring with IVF. The chance of this combination occurring in a spontaneous pregnancy is infinitesimal.

Sharing a placenta is not always an indication of identical twins. The two placentas of fraternal twins sometimes fuse together during pregnancy, as previously mentioned. Furthermore, identical twins will have separate placentas if the division of the embryo occurs within the first three days after fertilization. Such diamnionic, dichorionic identical twins represent 25 to 30 percent of identical twins. In natural conception two-thirds of identical twins have one chorion.

If the embryo division occurs between the fourth and eighth days after fertilization, the identical twins will share the same placenta and chorion, but each will have its own amnion. These twins are said to be diamnionic and monochorionic.

Joey and Harry are diamnionic, monochorionic twins who were recently born to a 39-year-old physician's assistant, the daughter of friends since medical school days over 50 years ago. She and her husband recognize subtle differences in the twin boys. She notes that "one has fuller cheeks and the other a slightly elongated head by comparison."

If the division of the embryo occurs between the eighth and twelfth day after fertilization, it is too late in development for separate amnions to form for each twin. This monoamnionic and monochorionic condition is dangerous, with a 50 percent risk of mortality. Fortunately, this condition is also rare, occurring in less than 2 percent of identical twins.

If division does not occur in the embryo until 13 to 15 days after fertilization, the separation cannot be completed, resulting in the twins remaining attached to one another. That is how conjoined twins typically develop. The degree to which the embryo splits and the timing of the split are believed to determine how and where the twins' bodies are joined. Some researchers believe the embryos of conjoined twins completely separate between the eighth and twelfth days after fertilization, but then reconnect between days 13 and 15. This is the so-called "fusion theory" of conjoined twin development. The competing "fission theory" proposes that incomplete division of the embryo 13 to 15 days after fertilization result in two growth centers that retain a connection at some point. Conjoined twins are monoamnionic and monochorionic. Only about 25 percent of conjoined twins survive pregnancy and delivery.

Mirror Image Twins

About 25 percent of identical twins are mirror images of one another—a phenomenon sometimes referred to as reversed asymmetry. Reversed asymmetry is reflected in certain physical characteristics, such as hair whorl patterns. If one mirror image twin has hair that grows in a clockwise orientation, the other twin typically has hair that grows in a counter-clockwise direction. The twins may also tend to part their hair on opposite sides. In some cases, mirror image twins may have birthmarks or dimples on the same part of their bodies but on opposite sides. Each twin may have left and right feet of different sizes, but one twin will have a larger left foot and the other twin a larger right foot. The twins may have a movement disorder in opposite (left or right) eyes. As children, they may lose their teeth in a mirror image pattern.

Some mirror image twins also demonstrate reversed asymmetry with one being right-handed and the other being left-handed. However, the reasons for this reversed asymmetry in handedness are complex and related to the handedness of their parents and their family, rather than to being mirror image twins. Opposite handedness in identical twins should not be used as the sole criterion for determining they are mirror image twins.

Each left-handed parent increases the probability of left-handedness in their children by 50 percent. When both parents are left-handed, the probability of having a left-handed child is doubled. Mothers of twins are almost twice as likely to be left-handed as are their own sisters, and fathers of twins are almost twice as likely to be left-handed as are their brothers. Twenty-two percent of both identical and fraternal twins are left-handed, compared to only 10 percent of singletons. Left-handedness is more commonly observed in fraternal twins simply because there are twice as many of them compared to identical twins. The tendency to be left-handed also occurs in siblings of identical and fraternal twins. In other words, twins and their families have an excess of left-handedness, compared to the general population. Both of my fraternal twin grandsons, Michael and William, are left-handed as are a paternal uncle, aunt and both boy-girl fraternal twin first-cousins. My father, their maternal great-grandfather, was left-handed.

In summary, left-handedness has nothing to do specifically with identical or fraternal twinning or, for that matter, mirror image identical twinning. Rather, left-handedness is more common among members of families in which there are twins of any kind, including the grandparents, mothers, fathers, sisters and brothers of twins. I suspect the phenomenon of handedness in twins has complex genetic linkages not precisely defined.

Is it possible the brains of mirror image twins have reversed asymmetry, with the functions of their left and right cerebral hemispheres being opposite? Brain research has shown that, although both sides of the brain are involved in most activities, the left side of the brain is where most mental processes related to language and logical thought occur, and the right side is where more visual and intuitive processes occur. Most people seem to have either a dominant right or left cerebral hemisphere, but the functions of the hemispheres are the same in all people. No association between cerebral hemisphere function and mirror image twins has been found.

It is commonly believed mirror image twins have finger, palm and heel prints that are mirror images of one another. But that belief is not true. The prints of any pair of identical twins are more alike than are the prints of two unrelated people, with a high correlation of loops, valleys, whorls and ridges. As with all identical twins, however, the details of hand and foot prints in mirror image twins are not identical—nor are they mirror images. Patterns on hands and feet appear to be related to mechanical, compressive forces each fetus experiences in the uterus. The patterns form as stresses develop in the skin between the epidermis (outer layer of skin) and dermis (inner layer of skin) at a crucial stage of development. These forces produce subtle but recognizable differences in prints between twins.

What causes mirror image twins to develop? It is sometimes reported that mirror image twins result when the division of the embryo occurs between the ninth and twelfth day after fertilization. However, if that were the case, then mirror image twins would have the same high risk of mortality as do other monoamnionic and monochorionic twins (as previously described)—and that is clearly not the case. My review of the pertinent medical literature prompts me to believe mirror imaging is a reality among some identical twins, but it has no relation to the number of days since fertilization. I suspect it relates to the axis of the embryo, along which the split takes place.

Rare Forms of Twins

There are rare reports of twins who do not conform to the traditionally accepted classification of either fraternal or identical. Virtually all fraternal twins are dichorionic, but there are six case reports of fraternal twins growing within a single chorion. All those cases involved women who were using ART, and the mechanism responsible for the cases has not been explained. Another unusual case, reported in 2007, involves a pair of conjoined twins in which one twin was male and the other female. That was the only known case of conjoined twins of opposite sexes.

Children of Identical Twins

If the two members of a pair of identical twins marry partners who are not twins, the children of these two different couples would be the genetic equivalent of half-brothers or half-sisters, rather than cousins. This phenomenon was illustrated in *The Patty Duke Show*, a television situation comedy that aired from 1963 to 1966. Duke played the parts of both a teenager and her "identical cousin" [a biologically inaccurate term]. The remarkable physical resemblance between the characters was explained by the fact their fathers were identical twin brothers. Lyrics in the show's theme song got the idea across:

But they're cousins, identical cousins all the way;
One pair of matching bookends, different as night and day.
Still, they're cousins, identical cousins and you'll find
They laugh alike, they walk alike, at times they even talk alike.
You can lose your mind when cousins are two of a kind.

Here is another remarkable fact: If a pair of identical twins marries another pair of identical twins, the children of the two couples would be the genetic equivalent of full siblings.

Twin Language

The sounds coming from the intercom in my grandsons' room, as well as Cindy Schiano's observation about her twins, tell me both identical and fraternal twins have a special twin language. Idioglossia is the term used for the unique language shared by members of identical and fraternal twins. As twins learn to talk, they mispronounce certain words (as do singletons). Members of twin pairs are often capable of recognizing and understanding the mispronounced words of their counterparts, and they also tend to mimic one another—making it seem as if they have their own secret language, which sounds like gibberish to others. However, this phenomenon is a normal part of cognitive and language development.

Twin Studies of Nature vs Nurture

Identical and fraternal twins have been the subjects of numerous studies conducted by social scientists, psychologists and geneticists who wish to determine the degree to which genetic influences (nature) and environmental influences (nurture) determine physical and mental characteristics, behaviors and disease states. In theory, comparing individuals in sets of identical and fraternal twins should enable researchers to separate genetic from environmental influences.

It cannot be assumed the environmental influences of identical twins and fraternal twins are comparable. Parents tend to treat identical twins more alike than they do fraternal twins, such as by dressing them alike and assuming they have identical tastes, interests and talents. These environmental influences would tend to contribute to greater similarity in identical twins' traits, regardless of genetic influences.

Another complicating factor in comparative twin studies is assortive mating, the tendency of people to marry other people who resemble them in intelligence, personality, attractiveness and other characteristics. Children of such similar parents would be more likely to receive identical genes for some traits than would children of dissimilar parents. This phenomenon could lead to exaggeration of the influence of genetic factors for fraternal twins, because the genetic similarities could be due to assortive mating rather than to fraternal twinning. Assortive mating would not affect studies of genetic similarity in identical twins, because those twins are almost genetically identical with or without the effects of assortive mating. In essence, the effects of assortive mating may cancel out the differences in studies comparing identical and fraternal twins.

It is widely assumed that because identical twins come from a single fertilized egg that splits in two, they must share the same genetic code—and, thus, any differences between them must be the result of environmental factors (such as different life experiences). Using this simplistic reasoning, comparing observable differences between identical twins and fraternal twins should reveal the extent to which their genes affect these differences—without having to directly analyze their genes. However, one must be aware of differences between anecdotal stories and scientific studies of twins.

To understand the various aspects of twinning, we need to delve into the complex world of human reproduction and genetics.

Reproductive Biology

The 46 chromosomes of a human being occur in all our body cells in 23 pairs. However, gametes (sperm cells and egg cells) have only one chromosome from each pair. Thus, 23 of our 46 chromosomes come from our mother's egg and 23 from our father's sperm. Once an egg is fertilized by a sperm (the moment of conception), it is called a zygote. A zygote—with the full complement of chromosomes—develops into an embryo, which becomes a fetus. These three terms—zygote, embryo and fetus—refer to an unborn baby.

Two chromosomes determine if the baby is male or female. These are called sex chromosomes. A female has two X chromosomes, one of which is derived from her father and the other from her mother. A male has an X chromosome and a Y chromosome, with the Y derived from his father and the X from his mother. Thus, the father's sperm determines the sex of the child. If the sperm cell that fertilizes the egg contains an X chromosome, the child will be female. If the sperm cell contains a Y chromosome, the child will be a male.

A closer look at the processes from the moment of conception (fertilization) reveals much about how a baby becomes a unique individual. Fertilization takes place in one of the mother's fallopian tubes. Immediately after fertilization, the zygote is referred to as being totipotent—meaning it has the ability to produce all the cells of the human body (the complete human organism). The embryo grows in size through the process of mitosis (cell division), in which two cells become four, four become eight, eight become sixteen, and so on. When cell division begins, the zygote is referred to as an embryo.

Approximately four days after fertilization, the embryo reaches the 16-cell stage. The embryo's cells are now referred to as being pluripotent—meaning each cell can give rise to many types of cells found in the human body, including cells as diverse as those in the brain, bone, heart and skin. These pluripotent cells are also known as embryonic stem cells (ESCs), the cells that are used in highly controversial research in which embryos are sacrificed to extract their ESCs. By definition, this type of research results in ending the life of a human embryo.

After the embryo leaves the fallopian tube, at about five to seven days after fertilization, it implants itself into the endometrium, the lining of the uterus. By day eight, each of the cells of the embryo has become specialized enough to develop into specific organs of the body. By the end of the eighth week after fertilization, the embryo is capable of motion, and the eyes, facial features and all other major body structures have begun to form. From this time until birth, the developing human being is called a fetus.

Genetics

Genotype is the name for our genetic makeup as represented by the DNA passed on to us when we began life as a fertilized egg. Our genotype comes from the contribution of genes from our father's sperm and our mother's ovum (egg). Phenotype is the name for the observable structure and function of our body and our behaviors. Phenotype is determined by our genotype, by environmental influences, and by the interaction between genes and environment.

The human genome is the complete set of human genetic information stored as a sequence of 3 billion pairs of nucleotides which are organized into DNA molecules. Nucleotides serve as the alphabet for the language of life and are represented by just four letters: A, C, G and T corresponding to adenine, cytosine, guanine and thymine. The nucleotide alphabet codes for the sequence of amino acids the body will use to build proteins. Heritable information is stored in DNA as sequences of these nucleotides that occur in numerous combinations, with the compound adenine (A) always paired with thymine (T), and guanine (G) always paired with cytosine (C) on opposite strands of DNA, creating the double helix. For this reason they are called base pairs. Combinations of three nucleotides indicate one of twenty possible amino acids. For example, CCT codes for the amino acid glycine so three sets of base pairs of nucleotides in different sequences form the gene for building an amino acid. Amino acids are the building blocks of proteins.

A segment of DNA molecule that codes for one complete protein is called a gene. A gene is a specific sequence of base pairs that occupies a specific location on a chromosome. There are 25,000 to 30,000 genes in the 46 chromosomes of a human being. Genes are located on chromosomes, which are made of long strands of deoxyribonucleic acid (DNA) tightly coiled around spool-like proteins called histones.

The embryo grows by cell division. To make new cells, an existing cell divides in two. But first it copies its DNA so that new cells will each have a complete set of genetic instructions. Cell sometimes make mistakes during the copying process called somatic mutations. The mutations, called copy errors, can occur early in the development of the fetus but because they are not in the sex chromosomes (X or Y) of the fetus, they cannot be passed on. They are expressed as a variation in the DNA sequence at particular locations called single nucleotide polymorphisms (SNPs, pronounced snips). SNPs can generate biological variation between identical twins by causing differences in the recipe for proteins written by the genes. The change could be in just one nucleotide of a base pair. These differences can influence a variety of traits such as appearance, disease susceptibility or response to drugs. Most SNPs were thought to arise after birth as twins have different life experiences and encounter different environments. Recently, they have been found to occur during fetal development with the average twin pair carrying 359 such genetic differences at birth.

The particular sequence of base pairs that make up genes—which are passed from parents to offspring—are the instructions for building and maintaining our body's cells. Those genetic instructions serve as codes for making proteins that, in turn, cause or influence the physical, psychological, behavioral and learning characteristics of individuals as well as predisposition to disease. Genes may undergo a process, called mutation, in which changes occur in their base sequences. These changes alter the proteins coded for by the base pair sequences. And the changed proteins then result in altered characteristics in the individual.

The mapping of the human genome—that is, determining the sequence of all the base pairs that make up the genetic code in humans—has led to the identification of the locations and functions of many genes. But has this genome mapping clarified the role of nature vs nature or shed light on the connection between genotype and phenotype? The answer is that analysis of the human genome has revealed more about what we don't know than about what we do know. It has shown us that most human traits are complex, with each aspect of cognitive ability, personality and physical appearance not being the product of single genes, but of the influence by multiple genes, multiple environmental factors, and interactions between genes and the environment.

Data comparing individuals from identical or fraternal twins who have been raised together or apart have been analyzed to determine the degree to which genes vs experience influence phenotype. Physical appearance can be affected by environmental influence, not just genetics—so that even identical twins can look different from one another. This fact can be explained by the concept of heritability, which is the extent to which an individual's genetic differences (genotype) contribute to differences in that individual's observed characteristics such as appearance

104

(phenotype). This extent can be quantified. For example, studies suggest 80 percent of an individual's height is due to genetic makeup, with the remaining 20 percent due to diet and other environmental influences. Academic research of the hereditability of intelligence quotient (IQ) provides estimates varying from 50 to 90 percent. The New York Times Magazine has listed 75 percent as a figure held by the majority of studies for the contribution of our genetic endowment to IQ, while 25 percent is influenced by environment and experience.

Thus, the same genotype—as in identical twins—can give rise to distinctive phenotypes. How do environmental factors cause such differences in phenotype despite similar genetic factors? The answers can be found in the developing science of epigenetics.

Epigenetics

The Greek prefix "epi" refers to features on top of or in addition to. Thus, epigenetic traits exist on top of or in addition to the traditional genetic basis for inheritance. Epigenetics is the study of heritable changes in gene function that occur in the embryo without changes in the DNA sequence of the genome. These epigenetic changes involve chemical reactions that influence how genes are expressed and whether genes are turned on or turned off. Epigenetic chemical reactions can occur as a result of environment influences, such as diet, smoking, and exposure to certain chemicals. Epigenetic changes bridge the gap between nature and nurture.

Methylation

One of the best-studied chemical reactions that result in epigenetic changes is methylation, in which methyl groups (molecules composed of one carbon and three hydrogen atoms) attach to the cytosine nucleotide on a gene. Too little methylation is associated with changing the gene's expression by turning it off and too much methylation turns it on. When the gene is turned off during embryo

105

development, the protein it codes for is not produced, and the metabolic activity carried out by the protein is not performed. This suppression of protein activity can have a profound impact on the form and function of cells, tissues and organs in the body. Conversely, if the gene is turned on at abnormal times during embryo development, the protein it codes for may be overexpressed, leading to metabolic problems. DNA methylation is a crucial epigenetic modification of the genome that is involved in regulating many cell processes. They include embryonic development, transcription, structure of chromosome material, X chromosome inactivation, stability of chromosomes and genomic imprinting (see below).

In July 2012, researchers at Australia's Murdoch Children's Research Institute reported that even in identical twins there are widespread differences in the epigenetic profile at birth. Studying chemical modification of DNA by methylation, they found that despite a common womb and amnion, the non-shared influence of the placenta and umbilical cord is different for each fetus observed at birth, with little change over their lifetime.

The B-complex vitamins, especially vitamin B9 (more commonly called folate or folic acid), act as methyl donors, making methyl groups available for methylation. It has been known for decades that deficiency of folate during pregnancy can alter an embryo's gene expression, resulting in failure of the neural tube to close—and a potentially life-threatening spinal defect in the baby called spina bifida. Avoiding the risk of spina bifida is the reason pregnant women are advised to take folic acid supplementation, especially during the first four weeks of pregnancy, when the embryo's neural tube is developing. Recently, mothers who used folic acid supplementation during the first month of pregnancy were found to have a 38 percent lower chance of having a child with autism or Asperger syndrome in California and 39 percent lower odds in Norway than those mothers who did not use the supplements.

Acetylation

Modification of histones—the spool-like proteins around which DNA coils, tightening or loosening to control gene expression—is another mechanism of epigenetic change. Histone modifications occur as part of a chemical reaction known as acetylation, in which acetyl is added to a segment of DNA. Acetyl is a chemical compound made of a methyl group bonded to a carbonyl group (composed of a carbon atom double-bonded to an oxygen atom).

The addition of acetyl causes histone changes that expand the DNA structure, allowing for genetic transcription to occur. Transcription involves making copies of the genetic code so that proteins can be produced from the code. Removal of acetyl causes histone changes that condense the DNA structure, thereby preventing transcription. Because these changes can affect protein production in the developing embryo by turning genes on or off, they can lead to major effects on phenotype. Histone acetylation appears to have a role in the development of atherosclerosis and diabetes mellitus.

Both methylation of DNA and acetylation of histones have been shown to accumulate in time. Older monozygotic twins were found to have larger differences in DNA methylation and histone acetylation, compared with younger twin pairs. These observations further support the assumption that methylation of DNA and acetylation of histones are influenced by environmental factors.

Genomic Imprinting

Epigenetic modifications that take place in the DNA of the egg or sperm prior to fertilization can be transferred into the DNA of the zygote after fertilization. When methylation that originates in the egg or sperm of a parent is transferred into the zygote, marking a chromosome as being inherited from that parent, this phenomenon is called genomic imprinting. Fraternal twins share fewer methylations than identical twins. In one study, researchers found age-dependent differences in genetic imprinting, methylation and histone acetylation among 113 pairs of monozygotic twins who demonstrated more of these chemical changes as they aged. This finding suggests increasing epigenetic differences over time may affect gene expression and, thus, phenotype without altering genotype. Furthermore, these epigenetic differences were greater in monozygotic pairs who had spent more time apart, suggesting the differences are influenced by environmental factors.

Each of the genes in the chromosomes of our body cells is represented by two copies, called alleles, one of which is inherited from the mother and the other from the father. In genomic imprinting, a gene inactivated (silenced) in the mother's genome as a result of increased methylation or decreased acetylation reactions is said to be maternally imprinted, so only the paternally derived allele is expressed in the offspring; and a gene inactivated in the father's genome because of increased methylation or decreased acetylation reactions is paternally imprinted, so only the maternally derived allele is expressed in the offspring. Imprinting is a dynamic process in which the imprinted gene (and the expression of the protein it codes for) can be erased and re-established from one generation to the next.

Epigenome

The distinct DNA patterns caused by methylation and histone acetylation reactions are like a second genome, called the epigenome. The epigenome regulates the activity of the genes in the genome. Think of the genome as the computer hardware and the epigenome as the software telling the computer when to work, how to work, and how much to work.

There are at least 210 types of cells in the human body, and each of these cell types is likely to have a different epigenome. All of the cells of our body contain the same genes, so why is one cell a skin cell and another a brain cell? The reason for this difference is that, despite having the same DNA, each cell type has a unique pattern of active genes and inactive genes as a result of that cell type's epigenome. During cellular division, the epigenome promotes the activity of some genes and suppresses the activity of other genes so that the correct cell type is created to fulfill a particular need of the body. The epigenome of skin cells promotes the development of more skin cells, while the epigenome of brain cells promotes the development of more brain cells.

Somehow, these complex processes are precisely coordinated and timed throughout an individual's body and life so that the fetus develops into a baby, the baby develops into an adult, and the adult's body continues to function throughout life. This constitutes one of the most profound wonders of biology, supporting, in my opinion, the concept of a divine designer of the human body (intelligent design) guiding the evolutionary process.

Epigenetic Inheritance

Epigenetic changes can pass from parent to offspring in a way that bypasses DNA—a phenomenon known as epigenetic inheritance. The changes are not necessarily permanent but can be passed down to at least one successive generation. For example, during the development of an embryo in the uterus, the growing organism is exposed to a wide range of particular environmental conditions, including certain temperatures, oxygen levels, sounds and chemical compounds in blood and other fluids. These intrauterine environmental factors can cause epigenetic changes in the embryo that affect its development long after birth—even during adult life and then passed down to his or her progeny.

Epigenetic modifications represent complex mechanisms linking genetics and the environment. These mechanisms not only bridge the gap between nature and nurture, but they show how the influences of nature and nurture work together to produce unique individuals. Family members, especially grandparents, tend to try to match up the appearances and mannerisms of children with that of other family members. They also tend to make predictions about the talents and future occupations of children. Epigenetics is the wild card that should prompt us to hedge our bets in these predictions.

Epigenetics and Identical Twins

Identical twins represent the perfect laboratory for studying epigenetics. Their genomes may be identical, but their epigenomes likely differ due to environmental influences. Their phenotypes are differently sculpted by epigenetic factors during their lifetimes, beginning with conception. Even in the womb, the individual embryos of the twins are exposed to somewhat different environmental influences. And these environmental influences become increasingly complex and divergent as the twins age, leading to distinct phenotypes, though the distinctions may be subtle. For example, some twins may have the same illness but at different times in their lives.

A study of 80 pairs of identical twins ranging in age from 3 to 74 showed 50-year-old twins had more than three times the epigenetic differences of 3-year-old twins. Twins who had lived apart for several years had the greatest epigenetic differences. Unlike twins' genetic profiles, the epigenetic profiles of twins are highly dynamic and changeable, resulting in identical twins who are not truly identical.

Contrary to popular belief, trained German shepherd police dogs can unerringly distinguish the difference in scent between identical twins. It is thought to be due to exposure to different infections. There is growing evidence that bacterial infections modulate epigenetics accounting for these individual differences.

The Second Code in DNA

In the December 13, 2013, issue of *Science,* researchers at the University of Washington reported having uncovered a second code hiding within DNA. This second code contains information that changes how scientists read the instructions contained in DNA and interpret mutations to make sense of health and disease. The genetic code uses a 64-letter alphabet called a codon. Some codons can have two meanings—one related to protein sequence and one related to gene control. In these duons, the protein-coding language is written on top of the language for gene control, hiding it. The discovery may open new doors in interpreting the differences between identical twins and whether they relate to this second code.

While growing up in Sioux City, Iowa, the Friedman identical mirror image twin sisters Esther Pauline and Pauline Esther were incredibly close. Both attended Central High School and Morningside College, where they both studied journalism and psychology. They wrote a joint gossip column for the college newspaper and both played the violin. Their marriages were a double ring ceremony on their birthday.

At the age of 37, Pauline began a writing career as Dear Abby, the advice columnist for a newspaper under the pen name of Abigail Van Buren. Pauline claimed that because she had applied for the columnist job without notifying her sister first, it created bad feelings between them for many years. A few months later, Esther began a competing personal advice column under the pen name, Ann Landers.

Ann Landers and Dear Abby each became a well-known newspaper advice columnist. Although the twins seemed to agree on almost everything they discussed in their columns for more than 40 years their styles differed. Ann Landers responded with homey detailed advice while Abby's replies were often flippant or risqué one-liners. In 1958, after only two years of writing their columns, they became, "the most widely read and most quoted women in the world," according to Life magazine. Ann Landers died at age 83 of multiple myeloma—a malignancy that begins in the antibody producing cells of the bone marrow, the plasma cells. Dear Abby died at age 94 of Alzheimer disease, which, according to her daughter, began at age 78. Their career similarities could have been the result of coincidence, sibling rivalry, genetics, family influence, business decisions, or any combination of these factors. It is tempting to speculate that Ann's death from multiple myeloma at age 83 and Abby succumbing to Alzheimer disease eleven years later, despite their "identical" DNA, may be due to a difference in their SNPs present since birth-or was it epigenetic changes that took place during their lifetime?

A final thought: Our genes do not program our destiny, but we all come with software from our family history that affects how we look, how we think, and how we behave.

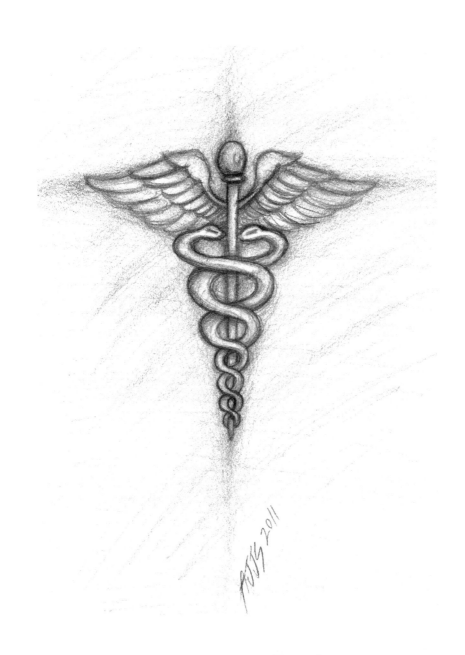

Separate but Equal

During the height of the Vietnam War, in the spring of 1967, I received a notice from my hometown draft board in Yonkers, New York. The notice directed me to report to Fort Wayne in Detroit for a physical examination and induction into the Armed Forces. At the time, I was 28 years old and doing my internship at Detroit

Osteopathic Hospital. The draft orders came as a result of the Military Selective Service Act of 1967, which was significant to me for two reasons: the act raised the age of general conscription from 18 to 25 years to 18 to 35 years, and it also, for the first time, allowed doctors of osteopathy (DOs) to be drafted into the Armed Forces as physicians. It was the first DO draft.

Since the fall of 1940—a year before the United States entered World War II—Congress had allowed osteopathic medical students to be deferred from military service until they graduated. Such a deferment had long been granted to allopathic (MD) medical students. The 1942 Military Appropriations Act, signed by President Franklin Delano Roosevelt, provided funding for "pay of interns in the Army Medical Department hospitals who are graduates of, or who have successfully completed at least four years of training in, reputable schools of medicine or osteopathy." President Roosevelt signed another appropriations bill in 1942 that authorized expenditures for the commissioning of DOs as Naval medical officers.

Despite these appropriations, osteopathic physicians were not included in the draft of the World War II era. Rather, it remained the policy of the U.S. Army and Navy that the only physicians to serve in the military were allopathic physicians—that is, MDs. The director of the Selective Service System at the time was Major General Lewis B. Hershey. Even though DOs were licensed to practice medicine in virtually all states, and many were residency-trained in the various branches of surgery as well as internal medicine, Hershey had decided the only place for osteopathic physicians and osteopathic surgeons was in the civilian war effort. Thus, DOs were given automatic deferments and were not drafted. The osteopathic medical profession considered the military's distinction between DOs and MDs to be an unfortunate form of professional discrimination.

The battle for equal rights of osteopathic physicians in the military began to make important progress in 1956, when Congress held hearings to consider a piece of legislation titled, "HR 483: An Act Providing for Appointment of Doctors of Osteopathy as Medical Officers in the Armed Services." The adversaries in these hearings were the American Osteopathic Association (AOA, the main professional group of DOs) versus the American Medical Association (AMA, the main professional group of MDs), as well as the secretary of defense versus the surgeons general of the Army, Navy and Air Force.

To understand the adversarial nature of the hearings on HR 483, some historical background is necessary. In 1951, the AMA, which had the authority to approve internships and residencies in military and civilian hospitals, became the dominant member of the Joint Commission on Accreditation of Hospitals—the accrediting body for military and civilian hospitals. The AMA's longstanding policy relegated osteopathic physicians to the status of cultists rather than real physicians on a par with MDs. According to the 1955 AMA Code of Ethics, no ethical MD could voluntarily associate with DOs. The Armed Forces' surgeons general bolstered this AMA policy by maintaining that allowing DOs into the Military Medical Corps would alienate the AMA and jeopardize accreditation of military hospitals. The surgeons general also feared DOs in the military would have a detrimental effect on MD recruitment, retention and morale.

Despite these objections, the legislation passed both the House and the Senate, and President Dwight D. Eisenhower signed HR 483 into law (Public Law 84-763) in July 1956. With the signing, President Eisenhower amended the Army-Navy-Public Health Service Procurement Act of 1947 by specifically recognizing the eligibility of DOs as commissioned medical officers appointed by the president with the advice and consent of the Senate. However, because the appointments were subject to qualifications prescribed by the secretaries of the Army, Navy and Air Force and because of opposition from the surgeons general, the Department of Defense could not implement the provisions of the new law for 10 years. During those 10 years, not only were DOs not drafted as physicians, they were not drafted at all.

In November 1961, two months into my first year as a medical student at the Chicago College of Osteopathy (now Midwestern University/Chicago College of Osteopathic Medicine), Deputy Assistant Secretary of Defense Frank B. Berry, MD, wrote the following response to the AOA's continuing request for implementation of Public Law 84-763: "While Doctors of Osteopathy are not presently being commissioned in the Medical Corps, by the same token neither are they being called up to fill requests for physicians which have recently been transmitted to the National Headquarters of Selective Service by the Defense Department." He further wrote, "...no osteopath will be called into the Armed Forces." Dr. Berry's main argument was that no DO commissions would be made because the Armed Forces' surgeons general had made no specific requests for osteopathic physicians to the Selective Service System.

By the mid-1960s, American participation in the Vietnam War had escalated and the need for military physicians had grown. In March 1966, the Camden County (New Jersey) Medical Society requested New Jersey Representative William Cahill to investigate the perceived unfairness of DOs being exempt from military service while MDs had been subject to the draft since World War I. In an address to the House of Representatives, Congressman Cahill said both his MD and DO constituents agreed DOs should be drafted into the Armed Forces. Cahill's probing prompted Secretary of Defense Robert McNamara, on May 3, 1966, to order the Military Medical Corps to accept qualified osteopathic physicians who volunteered for service. However, McNamara's order did not address active recruiting or drafting of DOs.

Several DOs volunteered for service in 1966. The first to volunteer was a 1965 graduate of the Kirksville College of Osteopathic

Medicine in Missouri—Harry J. Walter, DO, from Leawood, Kansas. Dr. Walter joined the Air Force on May 3, 1966—the very day the military announced it would accept DOs as physicians. He was sworn in on July 14, 1966, as a first lieutenant in the U.S. Air Force Medical Corps. Six months later, he was assigned to the 12th Air Force Hospital in Cam Ranh Bay, Vietnam, and was promoted to captain.

Andrew Lovy, OD, DO, a 1962 graduate of the Chicago College of Osteopathy, had been practicing family medicine for three years when he was drafted into the Army in 1966—though he received his draft notice from the Detroit Selective Service Board not as an osteopathic physician, but in his prior professional capacity as a doctor of optometry. Because DOs were newly eligible to serve as commissioned medical officers, Dr. Lovy petitioned the Army to allow him to serve as a physician instead. After completing his basic training, he was accepted into the Army's 101st Airborne Division. He completed his airborne training at Fort Benning, Georgia, and was assigned to a paratroop combat unit with the rank of captain. Dr. Lovy was awarded the Presidential Unit Citation, the Army Commendation Medal, the Air Medal, the Purple Heart and the Vietnam Gallantry Cross with Palm. Although he was drafted as a doctor of optometry, Dr. Lovy can rightfully claim the distinction of being the first DO drafted into the Army.

The drafting of DOs did not begin until July 1, 1967, with the enactment of the Military Selective Service Act of that year. Below the "ORDER TO REPORT FOR INDUCTION" on the Selective Service's preprinted stationery was typed-in, "Special Call No.41 Doctor of Osteopathy." A total of 1,130 physicians were drafted into the U.S. Armed Forces in 1967. The quota for DOs was set at 10 percent (113) of that number—though DOs represented only 6 percent of all physicians licensed in the United States at that time. This overrepresentation of DOs may be partly related to the fact that, for decades, roughly one-quarter of all the physicians licensed to practice in the United States have been citizens of foreign countries—and, thus, not eligible for U.S. military service. According to the Immigration Policy Center, in 2011, 27.3 percent of the 985,375 physicians (approximately 269,000) in the United States were immigrants. The DO quota for the 1967 draft had been negotiated by the AOA, AMA, Department of Defense, and Selective Service System based not on the number of DOs licensed in the nation, but on the number of DOs practicing in each state. This system was used to avoid an artificially high draft requirement for those states in which many DOs were licensed but not actually practicing. The quota system also protected osteopathic hospitals that might suffer a depletion of staff in states with few practicing DOs.

Basing the draft quota on the number of DOs practicing in a given state rather than the number licensed in that state created an unusual situation for potential draftees in Michigan. A disproportionate number of DOs were drafted from Michigan because of the high number of DOs practicing in the state. Osteopathic physicians had long been attracted to Michigan because of state laws that allowed DOs to administer medications and perform surgery since 1913. Michigan also had one of the nation's premier osteopathic hospitals—Detroit Osteopathic Hospital (DOH), which, along with Chicago Osteopathic Hospital, was a teaching facility for osteopathic medical students from the Chicago College of Osteopathy (CCO). Prior to graduation, fourth-year students from CCO obtained three months of training at DOH. The plurality of interns at DOH was drawn from CCO. Moreover, DOH provided residency training for half of all osteopathic specialists in the United States by the year 1967. Osteopathic physicians who received any of their training at DOH tended to remain in practice in Michigan.

I am a classic example of this migration-to-Michigan phenomenon. In the academic year of 1966-1967, 17 percent of the 405 students enrolled in all five colleges of osteopathic medicine in the United States were originally from Michigan, and 9 percent (including me) were from New York. Disproportionately fewer DO graduates returned to New York to practice because of the paucity of osteopathic hospitals and postgraduate training opportunities in that state. Although almost twice as many graduates of osteopathic medical schools were from Michigan compared to New York in 1966, almost four times as many DOs practiced in Michigan than in New York. Thus, the DO draft quota for Michigan was almost four times higher than for New York, resulting in 20 DO draftees and 3 DO volunteers being recruited from the Michigan draft boards and only 6 DO draftees from the New York draft boards.

In the Vietnam War era, the oldest physicians were drafted first. This policy was to ensure the most experienced physicians, especially orthopedic surgeons and general surgeons, would be available to treat combatants. At that time, physicians were registered by Selective Service as special registrants and eligible for the draft up to age 50. A male MD who was drafted as a special registrant could apply for a commission as an officer in the branch of his preference. Not so for DOs—who were assigned to the Army, Navy or Air Force according to the perceived needs of those medical corps. Also, rather than the oldest, the youngest DOs were drafted first.

The rationale for drafting the youngest DOs—and for excluding those DOs with prior military service or reserve status—was to ensure a DO would not outrank an MD. Thus, all DO draftees were drafted as general medical officers (GMOs), the lowest rung on the military's medical ladder.

A DO in the Vietnam era could not be drafted until completion of an osteopathic internship. At that time, some states, including Michigan, required an osteopathic internship for DO licensure, and other states, including New York, did not. Michigan had a separate licensing board for osteopathic physicians, while New York had a composite board for both MDs and DOs, who took the same examination and were issued identical state licenses. I became licensed to practice in New York only a few months into my internship at DOH. Because MD internships were not open to DOs, any DO draftee who did not complete an internship had to do so at an osteopathic institution before being inducted into the Armed Forces.

Deferments and postponements were granted by the Selective Service System's local draft boards and administrative offices, which were staffed by reservists. Medical advisory boards evaluated a physician's claim that he was essential to the community or to the profession. The medical advisory board for DOs consisted of one or two DOs designated by the AOA from each state.

I received a deferment from military service because the New York medical advisors in my home state, where I registered for Selective Service, deemed me essential to the osteopathic medical profession. Their decision was based on the fact I was the first DO to have been accepted into a fellowship in hematology, the subspecialty of internal medicine concerned with diseases of the blood and blood-forming organs. The fellowship, at the University of Washington School of Medicine in Seattle, was sponsored and supported by the Chicago College of Osteopathy.

Allopathic physicians had deferment options not available to osteopathic physicians as a result of the so-called Berry Plan, which was instituted in 1954 by Deputy Assistant Secretary of Defense, Berry, in response to complaints from the AMA, the Association of American Medical Colleges, and the American Hospital Association that the Korean War-era draft was depriving them of interns and residents. The Berry Plan allowed the youngest MDs to be deferred from military service while they acquired specialty training in civilian institutions. The plan gave the young MDs three options: enter the Armed Forces immediately after internship and return to residency after service; spend one year in residency after internship, then complete the residency after service; or enter the service after completing residency training in the specialty of their choice. The latter choice—which proved to be the most attractive option—permitted MDs to secure their residency, practice their specialty while in the service, and not be drafted until up to 20 years later.

Deferments for completing civilian residencies through the Berry Plan were not available to DOs. Military residencies were not open to DOs. Osteopathic physician draftees were not offered the branch of service of their choice. Obviously, the military continued to see DOs as less than equal to MDs.

The military made a major step toward recognizing the equality of DOs with MDs in June 1968, when the Army Medical Service was redesignated as the Army Medical Department. The new department's documents read, "The Medical Corp consists entirely of commissioned medical officers who are physicians (doctors of medicine and doctors of osteopathic medicine) who have completed at least one year of post-graduate training (internship)..." Then, in 1973, the Armed Forces were converted to an all-volunteer military, putting an end to the drafting of physicians along with the drafting of general registrants.

The requirement for men to register with Selective Service was suspended in 1975, and state and local draft boards and offices were closed the following year. In 1980, President Jimmy Carter directed the Selective Service to restart registration of male civilians between the ages of 18 and 25 in response to the Soviet invasion of Afghanistan—a requirement that continues today.
After decades of fighting for recognition of their equality with MDs, osteopathic physicians have distinguished themselves in the U.S. Armed Forces. Many members of the profession feel that the first DOs who served as military officers paved the way for the significant DO presence in the uniformed services. The ultimate sacrifice was made by James F. Sosnowski, DO, a 1965 graduate of the Des Moines (Iowa) University College of Osteopathic Medicine. He was killed on February 16, 1968—two weeks shy of

his 28th birthday. The makeshift field hospital near Tay Ninh, Vietnam, took a direct hit by a mortar shell while he was examining a soldier. Both he and the patient were killed instantly.

Today, there are 29 colleges of osteopathic medicine offering instruction on 37 campuses in 29 states. As of 2012, there were 82,500 osteopathic physicians in the United States—eight times the number when I graduated in 1966. Currently, more than 2,200 osteopathic physicians serve in the US Army, Navy, Air Force and Public Health Service. Although DOs represent only 6 percent of the total physician population in the United States, about 8 percent of all military physicians are osteopathic physicians. It is ironic the major antagonists to the first draft of DOs as physicians were the surgeons general of the Armed Forces. In October 1996—40 years after President Eisenhower signed Public Law 84-763—Lieutenant General Ronald R. Blanck, DO, MC, was appointed as the 39th surgeon general of the Army. He served in that capacity for four years. There is now complete parity for DOs and MDs in all branches of the military and public health services.

A final thought: Norman Schwarzkopf, United States Army General who served as the commander of the Coalition Forces in the Gulf War of 1991, said "The truth of the matter is that you always know the right thing to do. The hard part is doing it."

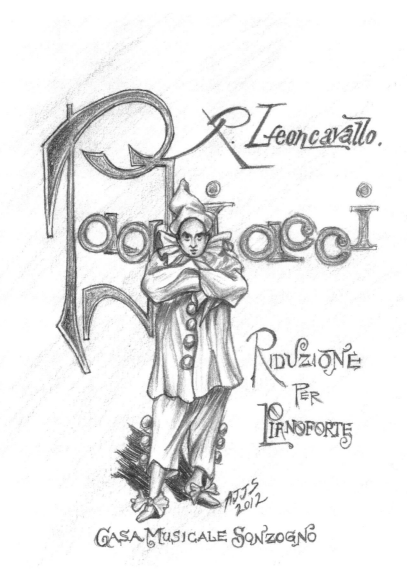

Humor as Medicine

Making jokes and laughing at others' jokes were responsible for most of the entries into my permanent record as determined by the presentation nuns at St. Frances of Rome parochial elementary school. My jokes meant I often had to stay after school in silent detention and serve as the courier for many sealed notes to my parents. To this day, I recall my father's oft-repeated admonition, "Don't be one of these pagliacci [clowns, in Italian] in school." My father, Augustine Vincent, was a contemporary of Enrico Caruso, the legendary tenor who was born near my father's birthplace in a province near Naples, Italy. Caruso sang the role of Pagliaccio in Ruggero Leoncavallo's opera, *I Pagliacci*.

Despite my father's warning, my clownish behavior persisted at Fordham Preparatory School, resulting in countless jugs, which consisted of walking briskly for about an hour around and through the quadrangle adjacent to Hughes Hall on the campus of Fordham University. Ironically, my most effective teacher at this Jesuit high school was Father Thomas Crowley, who embodied the Jesuit mantra to teach men for others. He regularly used humor to create rapport, cohesiveness and fraternalism, as well as to ease tension and get attention from the boys in class. In my senior year of college at Fordham University, I submitted a term paper on "The Theory of Humor." The paper, though representing only a modest effort on my part, managed to inflate my grade in a course titled Philosophical Psychology.

Somehow, I never could suppress my personality trait of employing humor to enhance interpersonal relationships. I made use of this trait in my more than three decades of medical practice in subspecialties that are not exactly a fertile source of jokes— medical oncology and hematology, involving the treatment of patients with cancer and serious blood diseases, most notably leukemia. As I look back on those years, I find I have developed a perspective on what constitutes humor as medicine, to whom it should be conveyed, how it should be delivered, and why it should be employed. I would like to share these thoughts with you in this chapter.

What is a Sense of Humor?

Some people possess a positive, skilled and adept sense of humor that enables them to generate jokes in a spontaneous, rather effortless manner in social settings. This is a rare gift. Individuals with this ability can easily elicit laughter from others and use humor to maintain and bolster relationships in various social settings and interactions.

There are two styles that fit the description of a person with a sense of humor. One style is self-serving, while the other style serves others. In the first style, an individual displays self-enhancing humor and a humorous outlook on life and can maintain this positive perspective even when faced with potentially stressful events and situations. These individuals also use humor as a coping strategy to minimize negative emotions and keep a realistic perspective on life. In the second style, the individual serves others by using humor as a type of medicine. This style of humor can be used to enhance interpersonal relationships. A physician can employ this kind of humor with patients to help identify and reduce concerns about health issues and then defuse those concerns through joking and banter. Such an approach is designed to reduce tension and facilitate relations with patients.

Is it irreverent and disrespectful to laugh and joke in the presence of a patient who is seriously ill? I do not think so, and I will tell you why. I believe a physician can be more effective in healing through the introduction of humor. Healthcare humor potentially narrows cultural and socioeconomic barriers. It relieves anxiety and can communicate useful messages. Healing is enhanced by providing an acceptable outlet for anger and frustration. Most of all, humor communicates caring.

Certainly, these goals can be accomplished without humor, but—for many patients—humor can serve as an effective therapy. Humor is a fundamental aspect of communication, a critical component of coping, and a vital source of comfort. Therapeutic humor is really an art form. However, it can also be approached as a science, within the context of the patient's illness and based on our knowledge of human nature.

Of course, you have to balance humor with sensitive listening, so that the patient understands you take their fears and concerns seriously. To me, it is a laudable task to create a receptive environment for patient-generated humor as well. By creating an atmosphere that fosters communication through humor, the physician is acknowledging that humor is a healing agent.

What is Humor?

Perhaps it would be helpful to clearly define humor in the context of healing. This is not an easy task, because humor is a broad concept that defies a good working definition. Most simplistically, humor is the stimulus and laughter is the response. But humor has various cognitive, emotional, behavioral, psychological and social aspects. Humor can refer to such stimuli as jokes, comedy films, cartoons and limericks; to such mental processes as the creation or perception of amusing incongruities and paradoxes; or to such responses as laughter and pleasurable feelings.

A sense of humor is a personality trait also difficult to define or measure, because it is highly individualized and modified by several variables, including age, ethnicity, education, political leanings, religious affiliation and emotional state. As a result of this variability, different people respond differently to humor. Getting the joke is not a product of automatic processing and does not allow for divided attention. A sense of humor can be thought of as a personality trait that relates to a regular (i.e., habitual) tendency to discover, create or appreciate humor. Having a sense of humor does not necessarily include the ability to amuse others—a much more difficult task. Very few of us can make a living as a professional comic.

The Importance of Laughter

Laughter is the most common, but not the only, behavioral response to a humorous experience. Although not a prerequisite, the ideal form of humor is that which provokes laughter. In the context of healthcare, humor is most effective when it is accompanied by laughter. The more you laugh the more benefits you obtain.

Laughter is also a social phenomenon. People are more likely to respond to a joke with laughter when they are with others than when they are alone. Laughter is distracting and captures our attention—much like a sneeze. Have you ever laughed even harder when you saw the way someone else was laughing at the same joke? Laughter can be infectious.

Is laughter medicine? Yes! There is sufficient evidence that laughter benefits both mental and physical health. This association can be explained by several physiologic and social mechanisms. One mechanism involves induction of a positive emotional state that accompanies laughter. Another mechanism has to do with stress modification. Humor can optimize an individual's strategies for coping with stress and increase social competence, resulting in improved interpersonal skills. In turn, the increased level of social support gained by the individual may confer stress-buffering and health-enhancing benefits. Laughter may contribute to the personal perception of better health or quality of life.

Laughter also exercises the heart and blood vessels. A belly laugh is like internal jogging—increasing the heart rate and stimulating circulation. Belly laughs relax the muscles by initiating contraction and reflex relaxation.

In addition, laughter exercises the respiratory system. Many of my patients who were using narcotics for cancer pain had trouble breathing deeply or coughing, putting them at risk for pneumonia. A few hearty laughs made their deep breathing easier and cleansed their lungs of secretions by causing them to fully exhale. Laughter is analgesic. During and shortly after laughter, an individual's pain threshold is raised and his or her pain is minimized—as reflected by a greater ability to endure pain, a decreased perception of pain, and reduced requests for pain-killing drugs. Some researchers have speculated that levels of endorphins, the body's natural pain killers, are increased by laughter, but this possibility has not been consistently validated. Nevertheless, laughter does appear to have an effect on the perception of pain by the central nervous system.

Laughing at a joke involves several parts of the brain. Using functional magnetic resonance imaging (fMRI), a medical imaging technology that measures brain activity by detecting changes in blood flow, researchers at the University of Rochester School of Medicine in New York searched for the center of humor appreciation in the brain. When study participants laughed at jokes they heard, fMRI images showed activity in the anterior supplemental motor area, a location near the top of the brain s associated with planning movement and initiation of speech. By contrast, when participants laughed at written jokes and cartoons— tasks that require a more complex comprehension of humor than listening to jokes—brain activity was most prominent in the ventromedial frontal lobe, an area associated with social and emotional judgment. The researchers found that all measurements of brain activity in response to all forms of humor showed activity in the nucleus accumbens, a small area at the base of the brain linked to pleasure and implicated as a key site in moderating drug addiction.

Although the ventromedial frontal lobe is likely the center for telling you what's funny, the accompanying laughter and feeling of mirth may be triggered by connections to other areas of the brain—areas involved in motor control (e.g., moving the mouth) and positive emotions. With the frontal lobe being essential to the appreciation of humor, the old adage is reinforced that "it is better to have a bottle in front of me than a frontal lobotomy."

What are the Specific Beneficial Health Effects of Humor?

It has been long held that individuals with a great sense of humor will have a longer life than the average person. Bob Hope and George Burns both lived to be 100. Sid Caesar, the king of scripted comedy, died at the age of 91 and Jonathan Winters lived to be 87. In March 2014, Carl Reiner was 92. Mel Brooks was 88 in June and Pat Cooper was 85 in July. Lucille Ball lived to age 78, Joan Rivers to 81 and Phyllis Diller to 95. Elaine May turned 82 in April 2014

I see a trend here despite the 2001 critical review by clinical psychologist Rod A. Martin of the University of Western Ontario, who concluded there was "little evidence for unique positive effects of humor and laughter on health-related variables." The variables measured by Martin included physiologic changes in musculoskeletal, cardiovascular, endocrine, immunologic and neural systems. He also found no evidence for pain-relieving or stress-reducing effects of humor and laughter, and no evidence for increased longevity among famous comedians, comedy writers and humor authors. In fact, he held that both professional humorists and serious entertainers died at a significantly younger age than did people who were famous for other reasons. Perhaps Martin profiled such comedians as Lenny Bruce, John Belushi, Andy Kaufman, Sam Kinison, John Candy or Chris Farley—some of whose premature deaths were accidental or related to drug abuse.

Martin's findings were a blow to my purposeful attempts to use humor as medicine in the more than three decades of my medical career. Nevertheless, his research has not diminished my conviction there is a medicinal role for humor and its attendant laughter—variables difficult to measure in the research setting, especially in the short term.

Still, I feel obligated to try to explain the discrepancies between my long-held beliefs and the findings reported by Martin. Perhaps the differences between my subjective observations and his more objective analyses may be attributed to the possibility professional humorists do not necessarily have a more humorous outlook, or use humor to reduce stresses, in their personal lives—even if they do relieve personal stresses among their fans. Alternatively, perhaps cheerful personalities are less concerned about health risks and do not take proper care of themselves compared to those whose gas tanks run low on cheerfulness. This would be the antithesis of the stereotypical hypochondriac whose prepaid gravestone was engraved with the epithet, "You see, I told you I was sick."

Martin claimed that even if you have a great sense of humor when all is going well in your life, you will be just as stressed out as the next person on your bad days. Importantly, he found that even if you generally find a lot of humor in everyday life, it doesn't help you cope with stress unless you make a conscious effort to actively use humor to deal with that stress.

In the final analysis, the recipient of laughter-producing humor may be the main beneficiary, rather than the one generating the humor. If that is the case, professional humorists are sacrificing themselves for others. I can live with that thought—no pun intended.

The ability to maintain a humorous outlook during periods of stress and anxiety is the acid test of an individual's sense of humor. It is unlikely humor that serves primarily as a defensive or denial mechanism would be conducive to effective coping strategies. More benign humor that involves perspective-taking or self-accepting aspects would be more relevant to maintaining mental health. Humor is so highly individualized and personalized that the future direction of research about humor and laughter should probably distinguish between styles or types of humor, including whether the humor styles are conducive to relationship satisfaction, reduction of interpersonal conflicts, empathy and intimacy—or whether the humor styles may interfere with social relationships. Researchers should also examine the impacts of humor on quality of life and mood improvement, even if a direct impact on mental and physical health cannot be measured by current methods.

A number of other research studies have suggested individuals with a better sense of humor have greater immunity to physical illness and experience fewer physical symptoms than other people. In the realm of psychological health or well-being, some studies have supported the proposal that individuals with a greater sense of humor have a more positive self-concept, with higher levels of self-esteem, fewer dysfunctional characteristics, and lower levels of stress, anxiety and depression. It has further been reported that people with a greater sense of humor derive more pleasure and satisfaction from the various social roles and life events they experience.

Jokes in Decline?

According to some humor experts, jokes are generally in decline. John Morreall, a professor of religion and humor at the College of William and Mary in Williamsburg, Virginia, has observed, "If you define jokes as fictional narratives that have a punch line, almost no stand-ups (i.e., stand-up comedians) do them anymore. They've turned instead to longer, observational, first-person stories that may not have punch lines." Witty banter and ironic commentary have largely replaced traditional jokes as the preferred form of humor. To the degree this newer form of humor is less belly-laugh provoking and more chuckle provoking, its therapeutic value is diminished.

Old-style joke telling had its heyday in the 1950s and 1960s. The jokes of that era were popular because they revealed little about the teller or the listener. They were clever, safe, and impersonal—such as the humor of Bob Hope ("Eisenhower admitted the budget can't be balanced and McCarthy says the Communists are taking over. You don't know what to worry about these days...whether the country will be overthrown or overdrawn"). Then there was the master of improvisation, Jonathan Winters, an admittedly bipolar comedian, described himself by saying, "I started out as an artist and what I do is verbal paintings." His characters, Maude Frickert, Ellwood P Suggins and the "100 year old man" were legendary in his 25 appearances on Jack Paar's *Tonight Show* from 1957 to 1962. Since then, people have become more emotionally open, to the point of wearing their hopes and hearts on their sleeves. This emotional openness has led to the popularity of jokes with a revealing, personal nature that may provide a window to the mindset of the teller.

At Sunday Services, the preacher was distracted by a young man in the back pew who held his head in his hands during the entire service. He appeared deeply anguished and upset. When the service was over the preacher approached the young man and asked him why he appeared so troubled.

The young man said "Reverend, I am 42 years old and still single. Every time that I bring a young lady home that I would like to marry, my mother does not like her. What can I do?"

"That's easy" said the cleric. "What you have to do is bring home someone who looks like your mother, dresses like your mother and acts like your mother.
The following Sunday, the young man is once again sitting in the last pew looking even more distressed. The preacher asked him, once again, what was troubling him.

He said, "I took your advice, Reverend. I brought home a girl who looked like my mother, dressed like my mother and acted like my mother. She even cooked like my mother"

"So what was the problem this time?"

"My father didn't like her."

One of the traditional reservoirs that has not dried up includes golf jokes. True, many of these jokes suffer from retelling and can be real groaners, but out on the course and in "19th holes" around the country golfers enjoy bringing them back to life. Most golf jokes revolve around frustration, obsession and the fickleness of the game. Golfers often feel little control over the outcomes of their actions and tend to laugh at themselves and their foibles on the greens. Many golf jokes concern lying, cheating, losing balls, throwing clubs and playing badly. Other golf jokes concern golf rules. Some jokes are disguised expressions of guilt about golfers abandoning their wives and family in favor of their beloved game.

God and St. Peter decide they must punish a priest who played hooky from saying Mass on Sunday to play golf. God lets the priest hit the shot of his life: a 410-yard hole-in-one. St. Peter asks, "Why did you do that?" God replies, "Who is he going to tell?"

Ray is about to chip onto the green at his golf club when a long funeral procession passes by. He stops in mid-swing, doffs his cap, closes his eyes, and bows in prayer. His playing companion, Dennis, is deeply impressed. "That's the most thoughtful and touching thing I've ever seen," he says. Ray replies, "Yeah, well, we were married 35 years."

During my last physical, my doctor asked me about my daily activity level so I described a typical day this way: "Yesterday afternoon, I waded along the edge of a lake, escaped from wild dogs in the heavy bush, marched up and down several rocky hills, stood in a patch of poison ivy, crawled out of quicksand and jumped away from an aggressive rattlesnake"

Inspired by my story, the doctor said "You must be some outdoorsman."

"No," I replied, "I'm just a crappy golfer."

The Ten Commandments

The Ten Commandments of joke-telling according to Paul McGhee, PhD, author of 15 books on humor, are:

1. Don't laugh at your own joke or story, especially in advance.

2. Don't try to tell jokes or stories that you don't know well.

3. Be sure the punch line is at the end. Don't telegraph what is coming.

4. Don't apologize if others don't laugh.

5. Don't try to explain the joke or story if people don't laugh.

6. Avoid put-down humor with groups of people. It's only a matter of time until you offend someone.

7. Be sensitive to the social situation. Know when any kind of humor or a particular kind of joke or story would be inappropriate or in bad taste.

8. Don't overdue puns. Remember puns are always funnier to the person who created them. Also remember that puns are funnier when you are under stress. So use them to take control of your mood by reducing the stress of the moment and creating a frame of mind conducive to maintaining a positive attitude all day long.

9. Remember that when telling personal stories or anecdotes, in some cases, you had to be there. Learn to anticipate the key information you need to communicate to make the humor fully understandable. Also learn to distinguish between those situations where you really did or did not need to be there.

10. Know when to stop joking and to become serious. Nothing is more frustrating than trying to communicate with someone who refuses to take you seriously.

Tried and True Tips

After his retirement, Deacon Don Lowe opened a mail-order bow-tie business, which is how I became acquainted with him. We chatted on several occasions, and I was flattered when he sent me a personalized and signed copy of his book, *Deacon Jokes a Pastor Can Tell*, published about 10 years ago. He passed away when he was in his 90s, but in his book he left a legacy of "tried and true tips to help you develop some good rules for becoming a pro at telling jokes":

1. You must be relaxed and sensitive to your audience

2. Always have a smile on your face. Take your time to elaborate every detail of the joke. Exaggerate a blow-by-blow description of the joke you are telling, using body language whenever you can.

3. Never, under any circumstances, make any racial or sexist slurs that could offend anyone. Also, don't make fun of a person who might have a disability (i.e., stuttering), and don't make fun of a person's religion.

4. The most important part of telling a joke is the punch line. You have to give the punch line everything you have. Pause for a few seconds so that the audience can anticipate the punch line and then deliver it with a slightly raised voice. At the end of the joke, laugh right along with your audience.

5. The final rule is an important one: Keep it clean.

I am confident the deacon would have approved these jokes:

It was Palm Sunday and, because of a sore throat, 5-year-old Johnny stayed home from church with a sitter. When the family returned home, they were carrying several palm branches. The boy asked what they were for.

"People placed them at Jesus' feet as he walked by."

"Wouldn't you know it," the boy fumed. "The one Sunday I don't go, he shows up."

One Easter morning as the minister was preaching, he reached into his bag of props and pulled out an egg. Pointing at the egg, he asked the children, "What's in here?"

"I know" a little boy exclaimed. "Pantyhose."

A little boy, in church for the first time, watched as the ushers passed around the offering plates. When they came near his pew, the boy said loudly, "Don't pay for me Daddy, I'm under five.

If I were to give advice to young physicians about using humor as medicine (which I have, on probably too many occasions), it would be to assess receptivity to humor before initiating any attempt at it. You have to make sure the anxiety and fear of a patient or family member do not exceed the threshold to appreciate your attempt at humor. Most importantly, be receptive to the patient's humor by listening to it, interpreting it and responding to its message.

For example, I entered the room of one of my patients who had just undergone a radical prostatectomy (removal of the prostate gland because of cancer) a few days before. When I asked him how he felt, he responded, "My sailing days are over, my harbor lights are out, what used to be my sex appeal is now my water spout." The message I got from this response was that the patient's main concern was he might have been rendered impotent by the procedure—a risk about which he had been warned. Alternatively, he may have been asking for Viagra samples (at a time when Pfizer Inc., the manufacturer, was allowed to provide samples for patient use without violating recently discovered ethical guidelines). Either way, the patient's humorous ditty opened up the doctor-patient dialogue that ensued.

Humor Types and Settings

A physician's attempts at humor can backfire with individuals of certain cultures who expect only reverence in the presence of a seriously ill person—and certainly in the presence of a dead body. Ethnic jokes may be successful in social settings if the joke teller is a member of the particular ethnic group mentioned in the joke. However, ethnic jokes are rarely useful in medical circles, especially if they disparage or ridicule. Also, if you can't do the accent, don't tell the joke, or else it will lose something in translation.

Humor as medicine cannot be aggressive. Such forms of humor as satire and irony can be amusing but seldom provoke laughter, and they have almost no role in therapy. Teasing, ridicule, sarcasm, cynicism and disparaging remarks to denigrate and put others down are not healing types of humor. Those types of humor are never useful because they disregard the potential negative impact on others, risk alienating the butt of the joke, and seriously impair social and interpersonal relationships. It is not funny to act like or be made to feel like a buffoon, fool or laughing stock.

Medical Humor

The compassion and caring of healthcare professionals leave us vulnerable to feelings of sympathy for those we serve. There is a significant difference between sympathy and empathy. Both arise from compassion and caring, but they relate to the suffering patient or family member in different ways. Sympathy allows us to feel another's pain as if it were our own. We feel frightened with them, angry with them, and depressed with them. Sympathy decreases our effectiveness as caregivers, because we lose our objectivity. Empathy, on the other hand, involves a detached concern. We can still express our compassion and caring, but without identifying with the patient's pain as if it were our own. Thus, we do not lose our objectivity and effectiveness.

Humor is a coping tool that can help provide physicians with a detached perspective. Caregivers often use humor as a means of maintaining some distance from the suffering, protecting us from a sympathetic response. Our ability to laugh serves as a release from the intensity of what can be an overwhelming situation. We may use humor to help us function in otherwise intolerable circumstances. However, our laughter—which is so therapeutic for the medical staff—may be perceived by patients or their family members as ill-timed, calloused or uncaring. Please understand that much of the stress healthcare workers suffer is the result of the fact we do care. We mean no disrespect. When I was once caught in a situation in which my laughter followed too closely on the heels of the loss of a patient, I used the words of Wayne Johnston's "To the Ones Left Behind."

"You saw me laugh after your father died. . .to you I must have appeared calloused and uncaring. . .Please understand, much of the stress health care workers suffer comes about because we do care. . .Sooner or later we will all laugh at the wrong time. I hope your father would understand, my laugh meant no disrespect, it was a grab at balance. I knew there was another patient who needed my full care and attention. My laugh was no less cleansing for me than your tears were for you."

Doctors, by nature and training, can read body language, and we are sensitive to clues about a person's sensibilities and limits. I try to use the kind of humor I sense patients will respond to or share with me. Some people need a more rugged and realistic type of humor. Everyone responds to a type of humor that points out the weakness of humanity, but shows no contempt and leaves no sting. We should not attempt to be comedians, especially the likes of contemporary professional entertainers who tell jokes or use satirical sketches and parodies to provoke laughter. Satire or parody are not consistent with the dignity of the medical professional and do not convey the healing power of therapeutic humor. Self-effacing jokes are fair game.

Self-Effacing Humor—Laugh at Yourself

As the doctor completed an examination of an alcoholic patient, he said, "I can't find a cause for your complaint. Frankly, I think that it is due to drinking."

"In that case," said the patient, "I'll come back when you're sober."

A gynecologist was a car buff but he never found the time to learn how to tear down and rebuild an engine. Upon his retirement, he enrolled in a trade school course on engine rebuilding. His first exam was to do precisely that. He received a grade of 150. Curious regarding why he got the extra 50 points, he questioned the instructor. "Well, you did a fine job in tearing down the engine, so I gave you the full 50 points. You did an even better job in putting it back together, so I gave you the full 50 points. As for the extra 50 points…I never saw it done through the tailpipe before, so I thought it was worth another 50."

Expressing frustration through humor communicates the message between patient and doctor, and between doctor and patient, without threatening the relationship. For example, upon entering the examining room where a middle-aged man was waiting for me, I said, "I apologize for the long wait before seeing you."

The patient's response was, "That's okay, doc. While I was in your waiting room, I got to hear about everybody else's illnesses and to give them my opinion. I'm thinking of accepting Medicare. In fact, I became eligible for Medicare while waiting."

That humorous response told me this person would be receptive to my own humor.

The hospital atmosphere for humor is trickier and more difficult than the office setting. During the acute stage of illness requiring hospitalization, when anxiety and stress are high, patients are typically not receptive to humor. Receptivity to humor is greatest during states of wellness and during convalescence. Since I was usually accompanied in the hospital by various combinations of medical students, interns, residents and fellows (collectively called house-staff), I found it important to keep the humor patient-centered—that is, to use jokes the patient could readily understand. Using inside jokes, such as medical humor meant for house-staff, in the presence of patients can hinder communication, increase anxiety and provoke anger among patients. Jokes aimed at the house-staff who share particular assumptions, experiences and contexts with the person telling the joke are very different than jokes aimed at patients. Patients may not see the humor or fail to find it funny because they are not in possession of crucial knowledge or insight held by the in-group.

How can you know when a certain form of humor will not work? This requires sensitivity to the human condition and an ability to read body language. When the situation involves excessive tension, anxiety or fear, attempts at humor have the potential to be experienced as inappropriate, not funny and even hurtful. Sadness, in and of itself, does not preclude humor. If an individual is mourning the death of a spouse after a long bout with cancer, he or she can often be comforted by a humorous anecdote about the lost loved one. For example, during the viewing in the funeral parlor, I related the following story to a man who had lost his wife to cancer:

Knowing your wife, when I recognized she was in the bargaining phase of dealing with her illness, I told her this vignette: A woman your age took her 5-year-old twin grandsons to the beach. As they made sandcastles, she dozed off under her umbrella. While she was sleeping, a huge wave dragged the children into the ocean. Upon awakening, she was devastated. Dropping to her knees, she prayed, "Oh God, if you save my grandsons, I will do whatever you ask of me. I will be very generous to the church. Please help!" Suddenly, a huge wave tossed the children back on the beach right at her feet. They were unhurt and giggling. They were alive and well. She looked to the heavens with her hands on her hips and said sharply, "You know, they were wearing hats."

I told the man his wife had gotten a chuckle out of it, as did he, attested to by a burst of laughter. He said, "That was just like her."

However, if the lost loved one's death was sudden, the spouse is likely coping with shock, fear of the future, anxiety and sadness. In that setting, humor is usually inappropriate.

Having encountered reactive depression in my patients with cancer on occasions too numerous to count, I felt comfortable recognizing and treating it, especially with humor. However, I was never comfortable when chronic depression was part of the patient's persona, pervading his or her life regardless of the nature of the underlying illness. The depression of such individuals seemed to be contagious to me, and it usually represented the low point of my day after their visits to my office.

It was my custom, as a teaching device, to have house-staff members who were spending rotations in my service to interview and examine my patients before I evaluated them personally. I usually directed these staff members to avoid seeing the seemingly humorless, chronically depressed personality types—thinking I was sparing the doctors in training. Then one day, unbeknown to me, a medical student entered the examining room of such a patient while I was still with another patient. When I finally went to that examining room, I heard the sounds of laughter and joviality as I approached the door. Upon entering, I was greeted by the patient saying to me, "This young doctor is hilarious. Why aren't you ever that way?" From then on, I no longer stereotyped such patients, and I attempted to inject a spirit of levity and mirth into the mix, along with a good dose of antidepressants.

Are There Gender Differences in Humor?

Forty eight percent of medical school graduates in 2011 were women but, collectively, the world of healthcare providers is dominated by women (61 percent of physician assistants, 91 percent of registered nurses, 92 percent of licensed practical nurses, 96 percent of nurse practitioners, 59 percent of nurse anesthetists, 90 percent of occupational and respiratory therapists, 95 percent of speech therapists and 74 percent of physical therapists). One might ask, "How does female humor differ from that of the male? Are women as capable of generating and appreciating humor as men? Are women as funny as men?"

Although male stand-up comics continue to outnumber female stand-ups, by about 2 to 1, an explosion in the number of female comics since about 2000 attests to a societal change in which humor has become more humanistic—giving more insight into the mindset of the humorist. Yes, it is very different from male humor. It is a distinct form of humor that arises from the experiences of women, and it serves distinct communicative functions associated those experiences. The stand-up comedy of Joan Rivers would be an example:

"I don't exercise. If God had wanted me to bend over, he would have put diamonds on the floor."

"I wish I had a twin, so I could know what I'd look like without plastic surgery."

"My face has more plastic than American Express."

Women tend to favor understatement, irony, and self-deprecation. They prefer word jokes, puns and shared observations. Unlike Joan Rivers, they tend to avoid one-line quips. Traditionally, women's humor is geared toward stories and real-life anecdotes. Researchers examining the scripts of male and female professional comedians found that only 12 percent of male scripts contained self-disparaging humor compared to 63 percent of female scripts.

It has been my observation that women in medicine use traditional one-on-one humor less often than do men in medicine. At the risk of sounding sexist, I believe many women find it difficult to initiate or generate humor. But this difficulty is not due to biologic predeterminism. Rather, it is a cultural phenomenon. Joke telling has traditionally been disproportionately a male activity, though social changes are now giving a new breed of woman the chance to express her innate sense of humor in the forum of alternative comedy. This movement, which began on the West Coast in the mid-1990s as an off-beat alternative to standard joke-telling, has led to a burgeoning number of female comediennes who poke fun at themselves and others, often with strong political and cultural undertones. An example would be the likes of Tina Fey, infamous (or famous, depending on your political perspective) for her mocking portrayal of former Republican vice presidential candidate Sarah Palin.

In contrast to men, women historically told few jokes in which they complained about the opposite sex, and they considered humor to be inappropriate if it entailed foul or sexist language. Now we are seeing a rising class of professional female comics who are just as vulgar and foul-mouthed as men, liberally sprinkling their humor with sexual innuendo and overt sexual overtones. A prime example would be Sarah Silverman. This new wave form of humor, in my opinion, has no use in any social setting—and, in the medical setting, would be detrimental to the healing process.

Senior Humor

I have observed that, with increasing age, people tend to become more receptive to humor. Perhaps this observation is a function of identifying with the senior audience, now that I'm a seasoned citizen. Despite aging being associated with loss of health, strength, vitality, social support and social meaning, one attribute not lost is a sense of humor.

Jacob, age 92, and Rebecca, age 89, are excited about their decision to get married. As they go for a stroll to discuss the wedding, they pass a drugstore. Jacob suggests they go in. He asks the man behind the counter, "Are you the owner?"

The pharmacist answers, "Yes."

Jacob: "Do you sell heart medication?"

Pharmacist: "Yes, we are a complete pharmacy."

Jacob: "Medicine for lumbago, osteoporosis and arthritis?"

Pharmacist: "All kinds."
Jacob: "How about hearing aids, denture supplies and reading glasses?"

Pharmacist: "Of course."

Jacob: "Medicine for memory?"

Pharmacist: "Absolutely."

Jacob: "What about vitamins and laxatives?"

Pharmacist: "Yes, a large variety."

Jacob: "Do you sell wheelchairs, walkers and canes?"

Pharmacist: "All kinds and sizes."

Jacob: "Great! We've decided to get married, and we would like to use this store as our bridal registry."

A tough old cowboy from South Texas counseled his grandson that if he wanted to live a long life, the secret was to sprinkle a pinch of gunpowder on his oatmeal every morning. The grandson did this, religiously, to the age of 103, when he died. He left behind 14 children, 30 grandchildren, 45 great-grandchildren, 25 great-great-grandchildren and a 15 foot crater where the crematorium used to be.

A gentleman in his mid-90s—very well dressed, hair well groomed, great looking suit, flower in his lapel, smelling slightly of a good aftershave, presenting a well looked-after image—walks into an upscale cocktail lounge. Seated at the bar is a nice-looking lady in her mid-80s. The gentleman walks over, sits alongside her, orders a drink, takes a sip, turns to her and asks, "So tell me, do I come here often?"

The type of humor the elderly are most receptive to is different than that enjoyed by the younger set. Seasoned citizens appreciate more one-to-one interaction, such as going to see in-person stand-up comics whose humor is contemporaneous with their own—rather than videotapes, audiotapes, comic books or comedy films. Compromised hearing and vision may have a lot to do with this being the case. However, videotapes of late comics whom seniors recall from decades ago may be appreciated. For the currently over-65 crowd, there is more laughter derived from videotapes of Johnny Carson and George Burns than from watching Jay Leno's monologues or hearing David Letterman's Top Ten List.

Much of the humor enjoyed by the elderly relates to issues of deterioration with which they are all too familiar.

Two elderly gentlemen were sitting on a park bench when one turned to the other and said, "Mac, I'm 83 and I'm full of aches and pains. You're about my age. How do you feel?"

Mac answers, "I feel like a newborn baby."

"Really? Like a newborn baby?"

"Yep, no hair, no teeth, and I think I just wet my pants."

A new wine has been developed exclusively for seniors. California vintners in the Napa Valley area, which primarily produces pinot blanc, pinot noir, and pinot grigio wines, have developed a new hybrid grape that acts as an anti-diuretic. It is expected to reduce the number of trips older people have to make to the bathroom during the night. The new wine is marketed as pino more.

In a South Florida newspaper was found the following senior's personal ad: MINT CONDITION: Male, 1932, high mileage, good condition, some hair, many new parts, including hip, knee, cornea, valves. Isn't in running condition, but walks well.

The senior citizen said, "I was always taught to respect my elders, but it is getting more difficult to find one."

Many seniors who have retired to Florida enjoy relating this parody when they recommend their choice to others:

You eat dinner at 4 o'clock in the afternoon.

All purchases include a coupon of some kind—even houses and cars.

Everyone can recommend an excellent dermatologist.

Road construction never ends anywhere in the state.

You don't have to take a vision test to get your driver's license.

This list is usually followed by the question, "What is driving like in Florida?"

Answer: "Well, at any time on I-95 or I-75, you will see a car in the left lane with the left blinker on. There are two hands gripping the wheel, with blue hair barely visible above the window level, and the car's doing 35 miles per hour."

A recent study has revealed alarming statistics that suggest senior citizens are the now biggest carriers of AIDS...hearing AIDS, seeing AIDS, chewing AIDS, bandAIDS, RolAIDS, walking AIDS, MedicAIDS, and government AIDS.

Jokes told by seniors are a kind of world commentary and are used as a tool to aid in coping with loss. Although the physician is bound to hear certain jokes repeated, seniors bring to the office an opportunity for the physician to show interest in their lives and to validate their continued importance as human beings as the sun slowly sets in the autumn of their lives—the so-called Golden Years.

Laugh at Yourself

We all laughed more as children than we do as adults. Perhaps we have lost the liveliness, joy and spontaneity we had when we were kids. We seem to take everything more seriously, including ourselves. The ability to laugh at your own flaws, weaknesses and blunders has long been recognized as a sign of maturity. But some children and adults just seem to have a temperament that allows them to laugh more than others when they find something that is funny to them.

During the 1992 U.S. presidential race, cartoonists were having a field day with Ross Perot's very prominent ears. But Perot captivated the hearts of the nation during a presidential debate when he said, spontaneously, "I am all ears." Like Perot, President Barack Obama made fun of his big ears one time during the 2008 election. While visiting Mount Rushmore, an adoring journalist asked Obama if he could imagine his face carved into the mountain someday. Obama answered, "I don't think my ears would fit. There's only so much rock up there."

It is said coincidence is God's way of staying anonymous. My horoscope on August 7, the day I started writing this section of my book, read, "Sagittarius (Nov. 22-Dec. 21): Jupiter changes directions in the skies today. Jupiter is the planet that reminds us that if you can't laugh at yourself first, then you have no business laughing at other people."

There is a liberating quality most people experience when they get to the point where they can laugh at themselves. However, many people have difficulty getting to that point. It is easy to see the humor in someone else's blunders or flaws, but it is another story when similar blunders or flaws occur in us. Yet, I believe the ability to laugh at yourself is a core component of a healthy sense of humor. Self-deprecating humor communicates empathy and acceptance of others' frailties and defects. When we find a way to laugh at our embarrassments, anxieties, frustrations and upsets, those problems lose their emotional grip on us and fade into the background. We feel at peace with the world, even though the world is embarrassing us at the moment. Those who cannot laugh at themselves and who have a tendency to take themselves too seriously are indicators of humorlessness.

The actor and comedian Steven Wright has developed the paraprosdokian to an art form with his dead-pan delivery of philosophical jokes. A paraprosdokian is a figure of speech in which, for humorous effect, the last part of a sentence or phrase is unexpected or surprising, causing the reader to reinterpret the first part. It is derived from two Greek words. We learned in the comedy film, "My Big Fat Greek Wedding," that all the words in our language are derived from the Greek. The word para means against and prosdokia means expectation. Some of his gems in this vein:

A clear conscience is usually a sign of a bad memory.

If everything seems to be going well, you have obviously overlooked something.

Everyone has a photographic memory; some just don't have film.

The problem with the gene pool is that there is no lifeguard. My gene pool needs some chlorine.

To steal ideas from one person is plagiarism; to steal from many is research.

My personal favorite: "He who laughs last probably didn't understand the joke.

People who can laugh at themselves tend to be cheerful, not overly serious people who are not strongly affected by negativity. How would you interpret the lyrics to the Bee Gees' song, "I Started a Joke"?

I started a joke, which started the whole world crying, but I didn't see that the joke was on me, oh no.

I started to cry, this started the whole world laughing, oh, if I had only seen that the joke was on me.

I looked at the skies, running my hands over my eyes, and I fell out of bed, hurting my head from things that I'd said.
Til I finally died, which started the whole world living, oh, if I'd only seen that the joke was on me?

I looked at the skies, running my hands over my eyes, and I fell out of bed, hurting my head from things that I'd said.

Til I finally died, which started the whole world living, oh, if I'd only seen that the joke was on me?

Gallows Humor

Humor is an important part of the traditional lifestyles of many cultures, helping people to cope with physically challenging environments and situations. It is also a device for passing on lessons learned from life experiences through a tradition of storytelling.

Such gallows humor is the epitome of using humor as a coping mechanism. As a type of medical humor, it can be seen as hostile, inappropriate or just plain sick by people who are outside the medical profession. Gallows humor acknowledges the disgusting, intolerable, frightening or painful aspects of a situation and attempts to transform that situation into something light-hearted, amusing or satirical. It is the kind of humor that arises out of precarious and dangerous life-threatening situations. It is a way of laughing in the face of death—a way of overcoming fears. It may even involve joking about death.

Most patients with cancer say they know it is important to keep a positive attitude and to try to keep some humor and laughter in their lives, but they can't seem to generate a mood or frame of mind that allows them to find anything to laugh at. Their sense of humor abandons them when they need it most. These patients are usually exhorted to "take one day at a time."

One terminally ill patient used a variation of that advice when he said, "I live each day as if it was the last day of my life because someday I will be right." Another patient, an 85-year-old woman whose cancer was in remission for 35 years, was asked to what she attributed her longevity. She responded, "To the fact that I haven't died!" Woody Allen once said, "I don't want to achieve immortality through my work. I want to achieve immortality through not dying."

As writers of their own lives, patients have the authority and ability to turn tragedies into comedies. Those who joke about the saddest or hardest elements of their illnesses may make the physician's job a lot easier.

Making fun of life-threatening, disastrous or terrifying situations fits the category of gallows humor. In his book, *Man's Search for Meaning*, containing descriptions of his experiences in Nazi death camps, Viktor Frankl elaborated about prisoners who cracked jokes regarding their horrible circumstances. He wrote, "Humor was another of the soul's weapons in the fight for self-preservation. It is well known that humor, more than anything else in the human makeup, can afford an aloofness and ability to rise above any situation even if for only a few seconds."

An exhausted daughter who was primary caregiver to her elderly mother once said to me, "Mom has Alzheimer disease. But on a positive note, she gets to meet new people every day, and they are all the same family members."

A pre-medical college student writes to her mother and father:

Dear Mom and Dad,

I am sorry I haven't written in so long, but my stationery was destroyed in the dormitory fire. I had to leap from my burning dorm room. My fall was broken by a boy who happened to be passing by on his motorcycle, but I had to be put in a body cast because of the fractures. I am now out of the hospital and have moved in with the boy who rescued me, since most of my things were destroyed in the fire. The doctors tell me they have to modify the body cast to accommodate my expanding uterus. I know you have always wanted a grandchild, so you will be pleased to know you will soon have one.

Love, Mary

PS. There was no fire. My health is perfectly fine, and I'm not pregnant. In fact, I do not even have a boyfriend. However, I did get a D in organic chemistry and a C in comparative anatomy. I just wanted to make sure you keep it all in perspective.

In a dark and hazy room, peering into a crystal ball, the gypsy fortune teller delivered grave news, "There's no easy way to tell you this, so I'll just be blunt. Prepare yourself to be a widow. Your husband will die a violent and horrible death this year."

Visibly shaken, Laura stared at the woman's lined face, then at the flickering candle, then down at her hands. She took a few deep breaths to compose herself and to stop her mind from racing. She simply had to know. She met the fortune teller's gaze, steadied her voice and asked: "Will I be acquitted?"

Doug Smith is on his deathbed and knows the end is near. His nurse, his wife, his daughter and two sons are at the bedside. In a weakened voice, almost a whisper, he says to them: "Bernie, I want you to take the Mayfair houses. Sybil, you take the apartments over in the east end. Jamie, I want you to take the offices over in the City Center. Sarah, my dear wife, please take all the residential buildings on the banks of the river."

The nurse is just blown away by all this, and as Doug slips away, she says, "Mrs. Smith, your husband must have been such a hard-working man to have accumulated all this property."

Sarah replies, "Property? He had a paper route."

You may have given some thought to why baby diapers have brand names such as "Luvs", "Huggies" and "Pampers" while diapers for old people are called "Depends." Here is the reason. When babies poop in their diapers, you are still gonna Luv'em, Hug'em and Pamper'em. When old people poop in their diapers, it "Depends" on who is in the will.

152

As his wife of almost 50 years maintained a vigil at the bedside of the dying man, he whispered, "Martha, you have been with me through all the bad times. When I got fired, you were there to support me. When my business failed, you were there. When I got shot, you were at my side. When we lost the house, you stayed with me. When my health started failing, you were there for me. You know what, Martha?"

"What dear?" she gently asked, smiling as her heart began to fill with warmth.

"I'm beginning to think that you're bad luck."

Some final thoughts: Physicians Eleanor Höfner and Hans-Ulrich Schachtner wrote in their 1995 treatise on humor in therapy, "One can learn humor as one can learn typing. Unfortunately, it is not taught in school but suppressed. It is important to educate ourselves in humor because it does not tolerate anger, hopelessness, and helplessness."

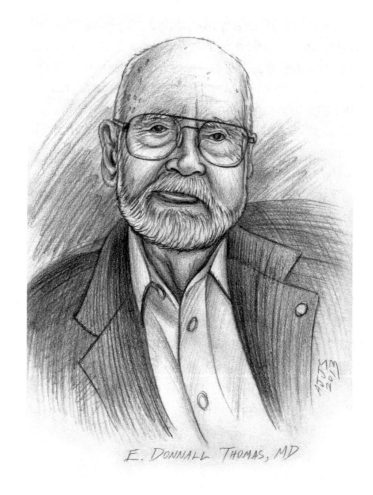

E. DONNALL THOMAS, MD

The Father of Bone Marrow Transplantation

I first met Dr. E. Donnall Thomas in July 1967 at the United States Public Health Service (USPHS) Hospital—also known as The Marine Hospital—on Beacon Hill in Seattle, Washington. He was the director of the bone marrow transplantation unit at that facility. The Marine Hospital was the first clinical rotation of my hematology fellowship among the five teaching affiliate hospitals of the University of Washington's medical school. I remember feeling honored that he subsequently remembered my name from the time of our initial introduction, calling me Augie. His commanding presence did not allow me to call him Don, as he was known to his friends and colleagues, despite the fact everyone else in the bone marrow transplant unit was on a first-name basis with him.

Dr. Thomas was a quiet and soft-spoken man who projected an aura of authority. When he spoke his carefully measured words, everybody listened. He was bashful and shy. Yet he was quite articulate during heated discussions with fellow researchers. Self-effacing, he was always quick to deflect praise from himself to the other members of his team. But he was a stern taskmaster and demanding critic who made sure deadlines were met for submission of scientific papers. He also made sure the papers were well written before he signed-off on them.

The hematology fellowship program required at least a 1-month rotation with the bone marrow transplantation unit. In 1969, I was privileged to be present when the team carried out its first bone marrow transplant using a matched sibling donor for acute leukemia. Recently, the more I've learned about his life, I've noticed many parallels between our careers in medicine and in life.

E. Donnall Thomas, MD, is known as the father of bone marrow transplantation. In 1990, at the age of 70, he shared the Nobel Prize in Physiology or Medicine with Joseph E Murray, MD. It is unusual for the Nobel Prize in Physiology or Medicine to be awarded to clinicians rather than to laboratory scientists. Thus, the granting of the award to doctors Thomas and Murray was interpreted by many as a special honor and acknowledgment of the importance of their work. In announcing the prize, the Nobel Assembly at the Karolinska Institute in Stockholm, Sweden, noted the discoveries by both men were "crucial for those tens of thousands of severely ill patients who either can be cured or given a decent life when other treatment methods are without success."

Dr. Thomas died of heart failure on October 20, 2012, at the age of 92. Dr. Murray's death soon followed, on November 26, 2012, when he was 93.

In 1956, Dr. Thomas successfully performed the first two human bone marrow transplantations on patients with uncontrolled acute leukemia. Leukemia can be thought of as cancer of the white blood cells. Acute leukemia progresses rapidly, while chronic leukemia develops slowly. The patients and donors for these first two bone marrow transplantations were identical twins. The recipients promptly recovered marrow function, and the leukemia disappeared. However, control of their disease was short-lived, lasting only six months.

Dr. Thomas and his team also completed the first successful bone marrow transplant from a tissue-compatible sibling donor in 1969. The 20-year-old woman, dying of acute leukemia, received the marrow from her sister. Twenty years later the recipient was alive and well. For the next eight years, bone marrow transplantation was limited to the 25 percent of patients with a matched family member. In 1977, Dr. Thomas' team was successful in performing the first matched transplant from an unrelated donor.

Dr. Murray pioneered solid organ transplantation, performing the first kidney transplant between identical twins on December 23, 1954. The patient had experienced end-stage kidney failure. The transplanted kidney began to work almost instantly. Both donor and recipient remained well. Dr. Murray made history again in 1962 by proving that kidneys from donors who are unrelated to recipients could be transplanted successfully if the donors and recipients are found to be compatible by tissue typing, and if the recipients are treated with drugs that suppress their immune system.

Don Thomas' life began in the sun-scorched farming town of Mart, Texas. His mother, Angie Hill Donnall, was a teacher. Don's father was a solo general practitioner who took him on house calls, initially with a horse and buggy. Don said, "I decided to go into medicine at the age of 5."

Thomas attended grade school in a one-room schoolhouse with a total of 20 students. His high school class in Coolidge, Texas, consisted of only 15 people. In his autobiography, he said, "I was not an outstanding student even in this small group." From there he entered the University of Texas in Austin in 1937. He had a modest start, earning "only B grades" until taking more difficult and challenging classes.

At the beginning of his second year, Thomas lost his father to an automobile accident. At that time, the nation was in the grip of the Great Depression. To support himself, Thomas waited tables in the girls' dormitory. In his junior year, he was leaving the dorm during a freak snowstorm in Austin when he was struck by a snowball, allegedly meant for someone else. It was thrown by freshman journalism student Dorothy (Dottie) Martin. "I naturally had to catch her and avenge the insult to my male ego," noted Thomas. They married upon her graduation two years later. Their marriage lasted 73 years.

Don received a BA in chemistry in 1941 and an MA in chemical engineering in 1943. He then joined the Army Specialized Training Program, receiving an Army Reserve commission. His goal of going to medical school came to fruition when he was accepted by Harvard Medical School, "thanks to Uncle Sam since the Army was paying for my education."

While Don was at Harvard, Dottie enrolled in a two-year medical technician program. In an interview she said it was "because it gave me an opportunity to spend more time with him but it also gave me a better grasp of what he was doing. And over the years, I moved from laboratory to administration and grant writing and earned my PhD in nagging." Dottie was Don's partner in every aspect of his professional life, from working in the laboratory to editing manuscripts and managing his research program. Known as "the mother of bone marrow transplantation," she died in her Seattle-area home January 9, 2015, at the age of 92.

Thomas completed a three-year wartime-accelerated program, receiving his MD degree in 1946. That was followed by a year of hematology internship under Dr. Clement Finch at Peter Bent Brigham Hospital. Dr. Finch was appointed the first chief of the division of hematology at Seattle's University of Washington (UW) in 1949. He retired in 1981.

Having served a postgraduate fellowship in hematology at UW under Dr. Finch from 1967 to 1970, I echo Dr. Thomas when he said, "Dr. Finch was a first-class mentor and he stimulated my interest in all aspects of clinical medicine, not just hematology." Dr. Finch's pervasive philosophy was to teach the teachers.

Thomas spent the next two years completing his army medical service at Madigan Army hospital at Fort Lewis near Tacoma, Washington, and in postwar Germany. His army service was followed by a year of postdoctoral research at the Massachusetts Institute of Technology and two years of medical residency at Peter Bent Brigham Hospital. This, too, is reminiscent of my anomalous career, which did not follow the conventional sequence of postgraduate medical education-internship, residency and fellowship, followed by specialized research. My career path sequence was osteopathic medical school, undergraduate teaching fellowship in pathology, internship, hematology fellowship, hematology research, medical residency and medical oncology fellowship.

In 1955, Dr. Thomas began his clinical research career at a teaching affiliate of Columbia University's medical school, Mary Imogene Bassett Hospital in Cooperstown, New York—home of the National Baseball Hall of Fame and Museum. It was there he carried out the world's first two bone marrow transplantations between identical twins. In 1957, he and his colleagues described their attempts to transplant bone marrow following high-dose total body irradiation in six patients. From the six unrelated donors, only one transient graft was observed to last for two to three months.

None of the patients lived more than 100 days. Compatibility between the patient's tissues (histocompatibility) was not understood at that time and no attempt was made to match donor and recipient.

Following Dr. Thomas' dismal experience with transplantation in humans, he returned to animal research, conducting experiments on beagles for the next 10 years. Beagles were probably chosen for several reasons. Like humans, dogs have marked differences in appearance, temperament and behavior (phenotypic diversity), though they are all descendants of a common ancestor (wolves). Beagles have a well-mixed gene pool with limited inbreeding. They are useful for research on cancers of the blood and blood-forming organs, because they have a propensity to develop non-Hodgkin lymphoma (a type of cancer of the cells of the immune system).

In 1963, Dr. Clement Finch and the famous endocrinologist Robert Williams, MD, author of a well-known textbook on endocrinology, invited Dr. Thomas to join the faculty of the University of Washington (UW) School Of Medicine in Seattle as chief of the division of oncology. Don established his research program at the United States Public Health Service (USPHS).

By the mid-1960s, Dr. Thomas had developed a system for matching the tissue types of his dogs. He demonstrated that irradiated dogs receiving marrow from matched littermates survived a long time. This concept of tissue compatibility among related donors and recipients prompted the idea of using tissue-matched human siblings in transplantations.

In 1972, the U.S. government closed the USPHS Hospital. After a two-year stint at Provident Hospital, Dr. Thomas moved his base of operations to the newly created Fred Hutchinson Cancer Research Center (the Hutch), and he headed the oncology divisions at both the Hutch and UW.

In 1975, Dr. Thomas published his results in treating 100 ill patients who had life expectancies measured in weeks. His results showed that 13 of the patients with otherwise incurable leukemia had, in fact, been cured through bone marrow transplantation with matched sibling donors. These results led to the use of transplants early in the course of leukemia while the patient's disease was in remission but with a high risk of relapse. Two years later, the team performed the first matched transplant from an unrelated donor at the Hutch in Seattle.

In 1979, Thomas reported curing half of the patients with leukemia who underwent transplantation with matched sibling donors when their diseases were in chemotherapy-induced remission.

Modern Bone Marrow Transplantation

Bone marrow produces all of the cells that are found in our blood: red blood cells that carry oxygen to all parts of the body; white blood cells of various types, including those in the immune system that help the body fight infection and cancers; and platelets that help blood clot and control bleeding. All of these cells develop from a type of precursor "mother" cell found in the marrow called a hematopoietic stem cell (HSC). The body is able to direct HSCs to develop into whatever different type of blood cells are needed at any given moment. Millions of blood cells are produced every hour in our body.

There are three sources for hematopoietic stem cells used for hematopoietic stem cell transplantation (HSCT): bone marrow, circulating (peripheral) blood and umbilical cord blood.

1. Bone Marrow Stem Cells

Bone marrow is the soft, spongy area inside the cavity of some of the larger bones of the body. Marrow produces all the cells found in the blood including red blood cells, white blood cells of several types and platelets. All these cells develop from the hematopoietic stem cells (HSCs) in the bone marrow. Since the 1990s, the "mobilizing" agent Neupogen (filgrastim) has been given to donors prior to the donation to increase the number of HSCs in the marrow. More recently, Mozobil (plerixafor) was added to give the HSCs extended capacity to repopulate the marrow with red blood cells, white blood cells and platelets. Possible adverse effects from these mobilizing agents include bone and muscle aches, headaches, fatigue, nausea, vomiting, diarrhea and difficulty in sleeping. These symptoms generally stop within two to three days after the last dose of the medications.

Obtaining bone marrow for transplantation is an outpatient surgical procedure that takes place in an operating room. The donor is usually discharged the same day or the following morning. The procedure requires general anesthesia, which puts the donor to sleep, or regional (spinal or epidural) anesthesia, which causes temporary loss of feeling below the waist. Common side effects of general anesthesia, which is chosen by 75 percent of donors, include sore throat caused by the breathing tube used in the procedure or mild nausea and vomiting. Common side effects of regional anesthesia are a decrease in blood pressure and headache.

Marrow is removed by multiple punctures with a hollow needle, which is inserted through the skin over the back of the pelvis bone. The area where the bone marrow was removed may feel stiff or sore for a few days, and the donor may feel tired. Uncommonly, there is bleeding at the collection sites. Because no more than 5 percent of the person's total marrow is removed, donating usually poses no problem with the donor's immune system or ability to make blood cells. The average amount of blood and bone marrow removed is about one quart, but less if the patient is a child or infant. The liquid is withdrawn from the bone and processed to remove blood and bone fragments. A preservative is added, and the marrow is frozen to keep the stem cells alive until they are needed. This technique is called cryopreservation. Stem cells can be cryopreserved for many years.

Most donors are back to their daily routines within three days after the procedure. The entire donation process may require a commitment of 30 to 40 hours over four to six weeks.

2. Peripheral Blood Stem Cells

Most HSCs stay in the marrow while they mature into blood cells that are released into the bloodstream. A small number of stem cells can be found in circulation, which allows them to be collected using a technique called leukapheresis (meaning removal of white blood cells). The same drugs (Neupogen and Mozobil) used to increase the number of stem cells in the bone marrow can be used to increase blood cell numbers in peripheral blood prior to donation. The stem cells are collected from circulating blood by leukapheresis several days after the last dose of the stimulating factors.

Leukapheresis does not require an anesthetic. A large bore needle, attached to plastic tubing, is inserted into a suitable vein in one arm. The only discomfort is the needle stick. The withdrawn blood is circulated through a cell separator machine that filters out and removes the stem cells. Simultaneously, the rest of the blood is returned to the donor through tubing attached to a needle placed in the opposite arm. Thus, the donor gets everything back minus the concentrated stem cells.

If the veins in the donor's arms are not large enough to accommodate the speed and volume of blood necessary for optimal operation of the leukapheresis machine, blood can be removed and replaced through a central venous catheter, in which there are two tubes (one for inflow and the other for outflow). This central line is placed in a large vein in the neck, chest or groin.

Harvesting stem cells by leukapheresis typically takes three to four hours.

During leukapheresis, the person may feel lightheadedness, chills, numbness around the lips and cramping in the hands. These symptoms are related to changes in the availability of calcium in the blood caused the anticoagulant blood thinner used to prevent the blood from clotting. They can be relieved by the addition of calcium to the donor's circulation. The blood thinner is the same one used to keep whole blood in the liquid state when collected by organizations like the Red Cross for blood transfusions. Some donors report a sense of euphoria during the leukapheresis. This is not totally understood, but could be partly due to the joy and fulfillment of knowing one may actually be saving someone's life. The harvested stem cells are cryopreserved until given to the patient.

Similar to the donation process for bone marrow, peripheral blood stem cell donation also takes about 30 to 40 hours out of the donor's normal routine over four to six weeks. But the less invasive procedure of leukapheresis, compared to bone marrow transplantation, has simplified the collection of HSCs. By eliminating the need for anesthesia and residual pain, leukapheresis has led to a dramatic increase in the number of donors worldwide. Approximately half of HSCTs are now performed using peripheral blood HSCs.

3. Umbilical Cord Stem Cells

After a baby is born and the umbilical cord has been cut, stem cells may be retrieved from umbilical cord blood and the placenta. This procedure poses no health risk to the mother or the child. Prior to the procedure, the mother must contact a cord blood bank, which will request she fill out a questionnaire and give a small blood sample.

Cord blood banks may be public or commercial. Public cord blood banks accept donations of cord blood at no charge, and provide the stem cells to matched individuals in their network. For more information about donating your newborn's cord blood, call 1-800-MARROW2 (1-800-627-7692) or visit Be The Match at www.marrow.org/HELP/Donate_Cord_Blood_Share_Life/index.html

Commercial blood banks charge a collection fee which can be $1,500 to $2,400 and the fee to store the cord blood is around $150 per year. Parents who choose this option are usually from families that have a history of, or close relatives with, diseases that may benefit from HSCT. Like bone marrow stem cells and peripheral blood stem cells, umbilical cord stem cells can also be cryopreserved for many years, but the actual shelf of cord blood is not known.

The Hematopoietic Stem Cell Transplantation (HSCT) Procedure

Before HSCT is performed, patients receive a high dose of chemotherapy to destroy all rapidly growing cells in their bone marrow—both cancerous and healthy cells, including HSCs. This conditioning, or preparative regimen, is an important element in the HSCT procedure. Its purpose is twofold—first, to provide adequate immune suppression to prevent rejection of the transplanted graft, and second, to eradicate the disease for which the transplant is being performed.

The destruction of HSCs results in irreversible loss of all blood cell production, including cells of the immune system, unless their production is restored by an infusion of healthy HSCs. This infusion is done through a central-line, plastic tubing inserted into a large vein inside the chest, usually the subclavian vein, which empties into the right side of the heart. Similar to a blood transfusion, the bone marrow, peripheral blood or umbilical cord cells are infused through this tubing. The HSCs travel to the bone marrow as if they have a homing device to their native land's most fertile field, where they can increase and multiply.

Within two or three weeks after entering the bloodstream and taking up residence in the bone marrow, the HSCs produce healthy, cancer-free red blood cells, platelets and white blood cells, including the cells of the immune system. Complete recovery of the immune system after HSCT may take several months for patients receiving their own healthy HSCs, called an autologous or auto transplant. Recovery may take from one to two years for patients receiving HSCs from donors, called an allogeneic or allo transplant. When HSCs are received from an identical twin, the HSCT is called a syngeneic transplant.

Human Leukocyte Antigens (HLA) and Organ Transplantation

The principle barrier to successful transplantation of HSCs is a group of genes on chromosome 6. These genes are responsible for the presence of proteins called human leukocyte antigens (HLAs) on the outer surfaces of the body's cells. HLA proteins are found on all cells in the body except the cells that make up the placenta. Their absence in the placenta is the reason a pregnant mother does not reject the unborn baby she is carrying, even though half of the HLA types of the fetus are different from her HLAs because they were inherited from the father. The identification of a person's HLAs is described as tissue typing or HLA-typing. Tissue typing revolutionized bone marrow and organ transplantation. The existence of the HLA system was first recognized in 1958, but it was not until 1964 that its importance in HSCT and organ transplantation was appreciated.

There are hundreds of different HLAs, but for purposes of tissue typing for HSCT, three groups must be matched between donor and recipient. They are HLA-A, HLA-B and HLA-DR. There are many types of HLA proteins within each of these three groups. Each has a numerical designation. For example, you may have HLA-A1, while someone else has HLA-A2. Some HLA proteins are common in the general population and some are rare. For this reason, an unrelated donor-recipient pair might have a 1 in 500 chance of matching or a 1 in a million chance, depending on the patient's specific HLA combination.

HLAs are inherited as a set of these three HLA groups—A, B and DR. Each set is known as a haplotype. A person's mother and father each have two distinct haplotypes on their chromosome 6. A child inherits two haplotypes from each parent. Thus, there are a total of four haplotype combinations you can receive from both parents. This results in a 25 percent chance of siblings inheriting the same two haplotypes. Siblings have a 25 percent chance of not inheriting any of the same two haplotypes, and a 50 percent chance of sharing one haplotype. The bottom line is that everyone has a 25 percent (1 in 4) chance of being an identical match to their siblings. Even if someone has four siblings, the chance of having a match does not increase more than 25 percent, since the odds are still one out of four for each sibling tested. That figure can be as high as 35 percent if there has been intermarriage between close relatives in the family, such as first cousins. Parents and children of the patient can also be tested, but their chances of being a suitable match are lower.

Matching donor and recipient for HLA-A, HLA-B and HLA-DR is an integral part of successful HSCT. The immune system uses HLAs to distinguish between one's own cells and foreign invaders, such as bacterial and viral infections, as well as cancerous cells. However, the HLAs can also recognize a mismatched organ transplant from another person, causing the transplant to be rejected. Mismatches of HLA-A or HLA-B increase the risk of rejecting the graft (the transplanted HSCs) and lower survival rates in recipients. But with HLA matching, graft rejection is now a rare complication that occurs in approximately 1 percent of bone marrow transplantations. In large part, this success is the result of chemotherapy or radiation the patients receive in preparation for HSCT. This pretreatment effectively eliminates the patient's immune system, allowing the patient to accept the immune system of the donor.

A mismatch between the donor and recipient's blood groups A, B and O can cause complications for bone marrow transplantation. Not only that, an ABO match can maximize survival from a HSCT. Selecting an ABO-matched donor instead of a major or minor ABO-mismatched donor significantly lowers the death rate. In a major mismatch, the recipient's immune system has antibodies against the donor's red cells that cause breakdown of the red cells in the donor marrow being administered. This is treated by removing the red cells from the donor marrow.

Success of the new marrow's ability to make red cells may be delayed owing to the recipient's immune system targeting the donor's developing red cells. This is often temporary but requires red cell transfusion for the recipient. In a minor mismatch, the donor's immune system is the culprit. Donor antibodies called isohemagglutinins from the infused marrow plasma can bind and destroy the recipient's red cells soon after the marrow is received. This can be prevented by removing the plasma from the donor's marrow. In addition, the lymphocytes (white cells that are part of the immune system) in the donor marrow can engraft and temporarily produce antibodies against the recipient's red cells. This is known as donor lymphocyte syndrome. Fortunately, this phenomenon is usually transient but requires careful monitoring and supportive care. After HSCT, the patient will have the donor's blood group and Rh type.

Because the patient now has the immune system of the donor, HLA mismatches can result in rejection of the recipient's tissues by the donor's HLAs. This rejection occurs in the form of graft-versus-host disease (GVHD), in which the donor's immune cells recognize the patient's tissue as foreign and attack the recipient's organs, leading to complications that can affect several parts of the body. The most commonly damaged organs are the skin, liver and intestines, resulting in such problems as skin rash, diarrhea and liver damage. GVHD may develop within the first 100 days (acute) or after 100 days (chronic).

GVHD is specific to HSCT and does not occur with transplants of solid organs, such as the kidney, liver, heart and lung, because they do not possess their own immune system, as does bone marrow. The transplanted bone marrow immune cells might still attack the recipient's tissues even if donor and recipient are HLA-identical, because the immune cells can recognize other differences between their tissues. When GVHD occurs, the patient must be given immunosuppressive medications, such as cortisone-like steroids and other anti-rejection agents, to lessen the degree of the rejection.

One study found that 54 percent of recipients of HSCT in which the donor was a female who had multiple pregnancies had a higher rate of chronic GVHD, compared to recipients who had male donors. This result was due to previous exposure of the mother to the foreign HLAs in her fetuses that were inherited from the father. Some cells from the fetus do find their way into their mother's blood during the course of a pregnancy.

A mismatch in HLA-DR increases the risk of the graft-versus-tumor (GVT) effect, also known as graft-versus-leukemia (GVL) effect. GVT is a response by the immune system of transplanted HSCs to the presence of the malignant cells that prompts the donor's transplanted immune system to recognize and attack the recipient's cancer cells. This condition is more prevalent among patients who received transplants for myeloid leukemia, compared to patients with lymphoblastic leukemia. GVT has not been demonstrated in patients with non-Hodgkin lymphoma.

The lack of this GVT effect was probably responsible for the short-lived control of acute leukemia in Dr. Thomas' first two bone marrow transplants in 1956. GVT is actually part of graft versus host disease. Because HSCT between identical twins causes no GVH, it does not confer the beneficial effect of GVT.

Age Limit for Recipients

The upper age limit at most centers is 50 to 55 years for an allogeneic (allo) transplant (related or unrelated) and 60 to 65 years for an autologous (auto) transplant. The decisions to place age limits on hematopoietic stem cell transplantation have been driven by higher complications and death in older age groups. This is attributed to their reduced ability to withstand high doses of chemotherapy (and sometimes irradiation) needed before the transplant, higher risk of short- and long-term complications of therapy and having other major health problems such as serious heart, lung, liver or kidney disease. The older transplant recipients also suffer acute and chronic graft versus host disease more frequently than their younger counterparts.

The phenomenon of the GVT effect in an allo transplant has given rise to the mini-transplant, otherwise known as transplant light. The mini may be the most important improvement in HSCT in recent history, opening the transplant door to patients who might not have otherwise been qualified for HSCT based on their advanced age or poor health.

The mini works by lowering required doses of chemotherapy and radiation prior to allo transplantation. This results in incomplete destruction of the HSCs in the recipient's marrow. While this approach increases the chance the cancer cells can survive the chemotherapy, it also preserves some natural immunity rather than leaving the patient completely defenseless. After the mini procedure, the donor's HSCs can still develop an immune response to the cancer—the GVT effect. The mini is usually better tolerated by patients because of the lower chemotherapy doses, making it a viable alternative for older patients and those in poor health. Moreover, patients' blood counts do not drop as low, because some of the patient's stem cells survive to make more blood cells. As might be expected, the trade-off of these benefits is a higher risk of cancer relapse due to incomplete eradication of the cancer cells.

In 2012, researchers at the Fred Hutchinson Cancer Research Center, where Dr. Thomas spent the bulk of his career after 1974, published the results of a number of clinical trials using the mini-transplant approach. Despite the mini being the last resort for most of the frail, high-risk patients, 35 percent of those receiving a mini were alive five years later. At the 2013 meeting of the American Society for Blood and Marrow Transplantation, it was reported that 55 percent of 56 consecutive but highly selected allo HSCT recipients, ranging in age from 70 to 76, who received reduced-intensity pre-transplant conditioning (mini-transplantation), were alive one year later. Forty two percent were still in remission with no evidence of progression of their acute leukemia or myelodysplastic syndrome.

The Three Types of Hematopoietic Stem Cell Transplantation

1. Autologous

In an autologous (auto) transplant, patients provide their own HSCs from their bone marrow or peripheral blood. Thus, they are reconstituting the cells produced by their own bone marrow and their own immune system. Because they receive their own HSCs, their immune system makes no attempt to reject the graft, and there is no risk of GVHD. However, because their own immune system is not active against malignant cells, any residual cancer cells left in the body (or any cancerous stem cells in the graft) could lead to relapse. Most auto transplants are performed on patients with multiple myeloma and lymphoma.

2. Syngeneic

A syngeneic transplant is received from an identical (monozygotic) twin. Because only 3 to 5 per 1,000 live births in the world are identical twins, rarely do patients who are candidates for HSCT have an identical twin as a potential donor. Since identical twins are exact HLA matches, recipients do not require post-transplant immunosuppression drugs, and GVHD will not develop. Compared to patients transplanted with HLA-matched but non-identical sibling donors, identical twin recipients are at a higher risk for relapse of the underlying malignant disease because the donor cells mount no immune attack—that is, there is no graft-versus-tumor effect.

3. Allogeneic

In an allogeneic (allo) transplantation, the patient receives HSCs from another person, most often a sibling or a matched unrelated donor. In 1977, a young patient with relapsed leukemia was admitted to the hospital where Dr. Thomas worked. The patient did not have a matched sibling. Dr. Thomas' staff was so supportive of his work that virtually all of them had been HLA-typed. One of the hematology technicians on the staff happened to have the same HLA type as the patient, and the technician volunteered to be the patient's marrow donor. The transplantation was successful until the leukemia recurred two years later. This event ushered in not only the use of an unrelated donor for the first time, but it made obvious the need for a registry of HLA-typed unrelated donors.

One of the advantages of an allo HSCT is that donor cells mount an immune attack and kill any residual malignant cells that had escaped the wrath of chemotherapy or radiation prior to the transplant. That is why fewer relapses occur after an allo transplant compared to auto or identical twin transplants, in which there is no graft-versus-tumor effect.

HSCs from umbilical cord and placental blood are considered forms of allogeneic stem cell transplant. Despite cord blood having a higher concentration of HSCs than is normally found in adult blood, only about 50 milliliters of HSCs are typically obtained from cord blood, making the cells most suitable for transplantation into small children. Newer techniques for expanding HSC numbers through certain laboratory techniques or the use of two donors have allowed cord blood to be used in adults. Using two sources of cord blood is possible, because infants' immune systems are immature, reducing the chance of tissue mismatches. A cord blood transplant can succeed even if there is greater disparity between the infant's HLA types and the recipient's HLA types than would be allowed with a bone marrow or peripheral blood stem cell transplant.

Transplantation deaths are primarily due to either GVHD or infection. GVHD damages multiple organs, making them more vulnerable to infection. Infection is more likely to occur with allogeneic transplants than with autologous or syngeneic transplants, because allo transplants invariably require suppression of the immune system with drugs.

Until the transplant takes, patients will need to receive antibiotics or antiviral medications to prevent or treat infections. They will also need to receive transfusions of platelets to prevent bleeding, and red blood cells to treat anemia. During this period, they will likely experience short-term side effects, such as nausea, vomiting, fatigue, loss of appetite, mouth sores, hair loss and skin reactions.

Potential long-term risks include complications of pre-transplant chemotherapy and radiation therapy, such as infertility (the inability to produce children); cataracts (clouding of the lens of the eye, causing loss of vision); secondary new cancers; and damage to the liver, kidneys, lungs and heart.

Many lives have been saved with HSCT, but with big rewards come big risks. Allogeneic transplantation can have a number of serious consequences, including death due to complications from the procedure itself. Thus, allogeneic transplantation may not be ideal as the initial treatment for most patients. There is a consensus among hematologists and oncologists that delaying allo transplantation for some diseases, including lymphomas, can give a patient the chance to benefit from conventional treatment and to enjoy a good quality of life until the conventional treatment ceases to be effective.

Hematopoietic Stem Cell Donation

Donor availability remains one of the major challenges to the success of allogeneic stem cell transplantation. HLA matching of a sibling or unrelated donor cannot be identified or mobilized in time for as many as half of patients.

In 2013, there were 69 HSC registries from 50 countries in Bone Marrow Donors Worldwide, a database headquartered in The Netherlands. Be The Match, the world's largest and most diverse registry of potential bone marrow, peripheral blood and donated umbilical cord HSCs, is operated by the National Marrow Donor Program (NMDP), a nonprofit organization based in Minneapolis, Minnesota. The NMDP matches patients with donors, educates healthcare professionals and conducts research.

Individuals never pay for donating and are never paid to donate. All medical costs for the donation procedure are covered by the NMDP or by the patient's medical insurance, as are travel expenses and other nonmedical costs. The only cost to the donor might be associated with time taken off from work. If complications related to the donation arise, the registry puts the donor in touch with healthcare organizations and doctors who are experts in the field of bone marrow and peripheral blood stem cell transplantation. Every donor who has such a complication is covered by a donor life, disability and medical insurance policy.

The NMDP maintains an international registry of volunteers who are willing to be donors for all sources of stem cells used in transplantation, including bone marrow, peripheral blood and umbilical cord blood. The registry currently records the preliminary HLA tissue types of 10.5 million potential donors and nearly 185,000 available cord blood units. On average, about one in 540 Be The Match registry members in the United States donate marrow or peripheral blood stem cells to patients. That chance of finding an unrelated matched donor is obviously related to the number of registered potential donors.

In 2012, more than 626,000 new potential donors joined the Be The Match registry, and its network of public cord banks recruited more than 20,800 cord blood units. In the United States, more than 5,800 marrow, peripheral blood and umbilical cord transplants occurred in 2012, an average of 490 transplants each month. There has been a steady growth in the number of transplants facilitated by NMDP averaging more than 10 percent annually for the past several years. However, it is estimated the number of potential hematopoietic stem cell transplant candidates in the United States alone is at least three times the number of recipients.

About 65,000 HSCTs were performed worldwide in 2012. More than 30,000 of those were peripheral blood stem cell transplants, 25,000 were bone marrow transplants, and 5,000 were umbilical cord stem cell transplants. About half of the transplants were allo transplants, with the other half being auto transplants. The cumulative number of HSCTs performed since Dr. Thomas began his work has surpassed 1 million.

Almost 30 percent of patients in need of HSCT can find an HLA-matched donor within their immediate family. The remaining 70 percent must try to find matches from Be The Match or other registries of unrelated volunteer donors. The NMDP website features a list of transplant centers that perform allogeneic transplants, including descriptions of the centers, survival statistics, research interests, pre-transplant costs, and contact information, as in:

National Marrow Donor Program
Suite 100
3001 Broadway Street, N.E.
Minneapolis, MN 55413-1753
Be The Match Registry: 1 612 627 7692 (or 1-800-MARROW-2)
Be The Match Patient Services: 1 888 999 6743
patientinfo@nmdp.org
http://www.bethematch.org

The criteria for a suitable donor of bone marrow or peripheral blood stem cells, according to the American Society of Clinical Oncology, are:

To be listed in the registry of the National Marrow Donor Program, potential donors must be healthy and between the age of 18 and 60. If matched with a person needing a transplant each donor must pass a medical examination and be infection-free before donating bone marrow. Most people taking medications can still donate bone marrow as long as they are healthy and any medical conditions they have are under control at the time of donation. Acceptable medications include birth control pills, thyroid medication, antihistamines, antibiotics, prescription eye drops and topical medications such as skin creams. Antianxiety and antidepressant drugs are allowed as long as the person's medical condition is under control. People who cannot donate bone marrow include pregnant women, users of intravenous drugs not prescribed by a doctor, people who have had a positive blood test for hepatitis B or hepatitis C, and those with specific medical conditions such as most types of cancer or certain heart conditions. People with Lyme disease, malaria, recent tattoos or piercings should wait at least a year before donating bone marrow.

Timing Is Crucial

Time is an important issue. It may take as long as six months to complete a search for a matched unrelated donor—primarily because of the lack of complete tissue-typing data for the entire donor population. The long search times make this time frame feasible only for those diseases with more protracted clinical courses, such as chronic myeloid leukemia, myelodysplastic syndromes and aplastic anemia. Searches for donors should be initiated early in the course of treatment of patients with high-risk leukemias. Most hematologists and medical oncologists believe allogeneic hematopoietic stem cell transplantation is now the standard of care for patients with acute myelogenous leukemia and acute lymphoblastic leukemia in first remission, as well as for patients with an advanced myelodysplastic syndrome or end-stage disease.

Decline to Donate

Forty-seven percent of Americans who are on donor registries say no when asked to donate. The anonymity of potential unrelated donors of bone marrow or peripheral blood stem cells makes it easier for the potential donor to back out if he or she is asked to donate. No one can be legally compelled to donate marrow or peripheral blood stem cells. A court case dating back to the 1970s helped set this precedent. In that case, a man had agreed to donate bone marrow to his cousin but backed out. The court refused to compel or force the donation.

Of course, there are many reasons why people may decide to decline to donate after they register. The informed consent forms presented to a potential donor can be intimidating and elicit considerable concern. A potential donor can easily balk after reading about all the potential adverse effects and the toxicity and complications of the agents used to stimulate the bone marrow to produce more HSCs for a bone marrow transplant. Other factors that may intimidate potential donors are the potential adverse effects and complications of leukapheresis and the need for general or regional anesthesia when procuring bone marrow.

Still other factors that may prevent donation are related to the changed health of the potential donor. He or she may have a condition that would be detrimental to the recipient if the donation proceeded. In addition, the potential donor may simply be unavailable during the sometimes very short time frame when the marrow or peripheral blood stem cells are needed. Furthermore, in a country with a mobile population, like the United States, many matched people in donor registries have moved and cannot be located when needed.

Age Limit for Donors

Many of us had our preliminary HLA type entered in a donor registry before the computer era, or we may have changed our e-mail addresses since registering. I was typed and registered with the NMDP as a potential donor 30 years ago. Now I am 74 years old and have aged out of the system. Patients especially need donors between the ages of 18 and 44. That is because younger donors produce more high-quality stem cells than do older donors. Age of the donor is the only trait significantly associated with overall and disease-free survival of the recipient. At five years after transplantation, according to the results of one study, the survival rate for the recipient was 33 percent if the donor was between ages 18 and 30 years; 29 percent if the donor was between 31 to 35 years; and 25 percent if the donor was older than 45 years. However, anyone between the ages of 18 and 60 can join the NMDP registry.

Making a Successful Match

If a match cannot be identified within the patient's family or in a registry, a match can be sought through a donor drive. The best chance of finding an unrelated HSC match is within the patient's ethnic and racial group. That is why donor drives are often held at ethnic churches, such as Greek Orthodox or Armenian Apostolic churches and such traditionally African-American churches as Southern Baptist or African Methodist Episcopal. People belonging to minority populations are increasingly underrepresented in donor registries and, therefore, have less chance of finding HLA- matched HSCs compared with the white population. African-Americans, American Indians, Alaskan natives, Asians, Hispanics and native Hawaiians and Pacific islanders are urgently needed as donors.

When I joined the registry, a blood sample was taken and I was typed for HLA-A and HLA-B. I am one of about 1.6 million potential donors functionally inactive because 99 percent of all transplants the NMDP facilitates use a donor selected from an HLA-A, HLA-B and DRB1-typed pool. They are identified from a buccal swab sample for DNA-based testing rather than a blood sample. (Buccal is the term for the cheeks or the mouth cavity.) The cells obtained from the swab provide DNA for HLA testing. Using a different swab each time and with the same pressure of typical tooth brushing, a swab is taken from four different sites inside the cheeks—top left; bottom left; top right and bottom right. Two swabs are used for initial HLA testing and two are stored for additional HLA testing when needed. After the DNA is extracted from the swab, the swab is thrown away. If you decide to remove your name from the donor registry, your remaining swabs will be discarded.

The method for collecting DNA is similar to what is seen on TV programs such as *Law and Order*. However, the NMDP uses the DNA only for HLA testing to determine an individual's tissue type. All new members are tested for six HLA markers when they join. If several potential donors are found to be a possible match, they are called for further high-resolution testing to find the donor who matches at a detailed level. The ideal donor is an under-40 adult male HLA matched for 12 markers.

Cost

The NMDP covers the cost of tissue typing for donors age 18 to 44. Those between 45 and 60 who wish to join the registry can do so for a tax deductible $100 payment. One transplant center provides donor typing free for immediate family members and a fee of $60 for extended family members and friends. If part of a donor drive for a specific recipient, a community or church group may pick up the tab or provide financial assistance. After a donor has been identified as a match for a patient, all costs pertaining to the retrieval of bone marrow or peripheral blood are usually covered by the patient's medical insurance. The total cost for the procedure can easily reach $100,000 or more for an autologous transplant and $200,000 or more for an allogeneic transplant.

Knowing the Outcome

Most donors would, naturally, want to know the fate of the recipient of their HSC donation. Some transplant centers may provide a donor with up to three updates on the recipient's condition within the first year after transplant. During that year, some centers allow anonymous contact between patient and donor. Some centers even allow direct contact between recipient and donor, with mutual consent, one or more years after the transplant. Such contact creates a potential for psychological trauma for the donor, similar to post-traumatic stress disorder, if the patient does not survive.

The reason for a patient's failure to survive may be unrelated to the donation. Perhaps the patient's body could not withstand the pre-transplant chemotherapy. The patient may have suffered an overwhelming infection before the marrow could take. Any number of complications could have arisen despite successful acceptance of the graft. Any feelings of unwarranted guilt or depression by the donor could be relieved with counseling, which is available through the registry.

Transplantation survival rates vary dramatically depending on the patient's age, disease type, stage of disease, type of transplantation and type of donor cells. Cancer type is one of the most important factors that determine which kind of transplantation will most benefit a patient. That decision-making process is Dr. Don Thomas' greatest legacy.

A Recipient's Experience

Upon graduation from the Chicago College of Osteopathy, the newly minted Lawrence Usher, DO, created a bucket list of things he planned to do before he died. He saw himself as one who sought adventure and living on the edge. The list went unfulfilled during the demands of his internship. Nor did he foresee that, in 1967, he would be one of the first osteopathic physicians drafted into the Navy.

For the first six months, Doctor Usher served in the field with the 1st Medical Battalion—a unit of the United States Marine Corps operated by the United States Navy. This unit provided medical support to the 3,500 Marines stationed in Da Nang, Vietnam, near its hotly contested air base. This was followed by six months as a general medical officer, triaging and treating Marine casualties. Living at the edge of an air base in the northeast coastal area of the Republic of Vietnam, about 85 miles south of the demilitarized zone, was likely not exactly what he had in mind by living on the edge.

From Usher's base, he could see the plumes of the defoliant Agent Orange being sprayed by low-flying aircraft and helicopters. The chemical itself had no color. The name refers to the orange-colored stripes painted on the 55 gallon barrels in which it was shipped to identify its contents. The aim of the spraying program was to destroy the cover provided by the jungle-like forest, depriving the guerillas of food and clearing sensitive areas such as around the perimeter of the base. Agent Orange is a 50-50 mixture of 2, 4, 5-trichlorophenoxyacetic and 2, 4-dichlorophenoxyacetic acid—considered low toxicity agents to humans. However, the manufacturing process contaminates the chemical with a dioxin which is a carcinogen—an agent directly involved in causing cancer. These chemicals were then mixed with kerosene, diesel fuel or jet fuel.

Following Usher's discharge from the service he embarked on a clinical career serving residents of nursing homes and extended care facilities. During the next 41 years he managed to run through virtually all the items on his bucket list. He commuted between the health care facilities in his charge on a motorcycle, skied the big slopes in Colorado, Utah and the Swiss Alps, lake fishing in Canada and Alaska and piloting his own single engine Cessna. Summers were filled with water-skiing, hang-gliding and para-sailing. Scuba diving found him in all the most exotic sites in the Caribbean, the uninhabited Cocos Island 340 miles from the Pacific shore of Costa Rica, the western Pacific such as the Republic of Palau in Micronesia, Yap Island in the Carolines, the Marshall and Solomon islands and the Philippines. He completed 316 parachute jumps.

In 1988, while skiing in the Swiss Alps, he experienced unusual shortness of breath while ascending a small incline to the ski lift. Upon his return to the Detroit area, he was found to be anemic. A bone marrow biopsy revealed that his marrow was replaced with scar tissue called fibrosis. A diagnosis of primary myelofibrosis, literally marrow fibrosis of unknown cause, was rendered. This entity is in the family of myeloproliferative disorders, a type of marrow cancer. Although primary myelofibrosis is not on the U.S Department of Veterans Affairs list of presumptive diseases associated with Agent Orange, the doctor is convinced it should be.

For the next five years, Larry was prescribed a cocktail of multiple vitamins and weekly injections of a testosterone derivative to maintain his hemoglobin levels to the point where he functioned well enough to engage in his usual level of professional and social activities. But by the fall of 1993, he required regular transfusions of red cells. Bone marrow transplantation was advised. Tissue typing of his three sisters and one brother failed to find a match. The marrow donor registry identified an unrelated 39-year-old male of his same Ashkenazi Jewish ethnicity as a suitable donor. He underwent bone marrow transplantation in Detroit on May 2, 1994. At that time, he was told he was the oldest bone marrow recipient from an unrelated donor in the world—at the age of 54.

Engraftment was successful unusually early. The marrow graft began making blood cells within a week. His only complication was thrush, a yeast infection, in his mouth. For almost a year, he required the immune suppressant, cyclosporine, to prevent graft versus host disease. The only visible signs of GVHD today are dry skin and patches of scalp hair loss. He continues to be treated for gout which predated his transplant and has a mild degree of inability of his kidneys to process protein, prompting a restricted diet.

Larry continues to punch his bucket list card as vigorously as before the marrow transplantation. When I interviewed him, he had just returned from a fishing trip in Canada. I asked him what advice he would give a person who is a candidate for a hematopoietic stem cell transplant. He said, "Just do it! There is no alternative. This is your only chance for life. I have had almost 20 great years that I would not have otherwise had."

A Donor's Experience

In June 2012, Robin Roberts—the fifty-two-year-old host on *Good Morning America*—told the world she was suffering from one of the myelodysplastic syndromes (MDS). With this type of marrow cancer, the bone marrow loses its ability to produce enough mature white blood cells to fight infection, red cells to transport oxygen to different parts of the body and platelets to prevent bleeding. MDS can progress to acute leukemia. Robin had been declared free of breast cancer five years prior with the help of chemotherapy administered as a preventative for recurrence of the disease. Although a rare occurrence, her MDS was considered to be caused by that same chemotherapy. Moreover, when acute leukemia develops from MDS it is usually resistant to further chemotherapy. For this reason she was considered a candidate for bone marrow transplantation.

Fortunate to have a sister who was an HLA match, Robin had a successful transplant in September 2012. She encouraged her viewers to consider being a donor of bone marrow or peripheral blood stem cells (PBSCs) to someone who might not be as fortunate as she was in having a matched sibling and would need an unrelated donor. They could do so by signing up on the donor registry at BeTheMatch.org.

Michelle Thornbury was one of those inspired viewers. Her decision to donate was made because of the loss of several family members to cancer. This would be her opportunity help in the fight against cancer. Within two weeks of signing up online, she was sent a test kit in the mail. It contained four swabs which she used to swab four quadrants of the inside of her cheeks—all while sitting on her living room couch. She mailed them to a laboratory in a prepaid envelope.

Five months later, Michelle received a phone call, followed by an e-mail, informing her she was a preliminary match. Further blood tests were drawn to confirm the match at a nearby university medical center to which she was directed by the National Marrow Donor Program. Michelle related that, "The ease of the matching process was an important part of how I wound up on the registry and became a donor eight months later." From the start, Michelle was assigned a personal representative from a regional blood center who guided her through the process. She described her support team as kind, sensitive and encouraging and was especially touched by nurses willing to talk about faith and prayer. Each time she was asked, "Why are you doing this?" by well-intentioned friends, she responded that it was "because it is what I was told to do" (by God).

Six weeks after determining she was a suitable match, Michelle donated her PBSCs by leukapheresis. The recipient's team preferred a donation of bone marrow over PBSCs but did give her a choice. Her doctor determined she was not a good candidate for marrow donation for medical reasons and advised a stem cell donation.

Despite great curiosity about her recipient, Michelle was given "only tidbits of information" because of privacy regulations. She was told "he is in a time zone which is a day ahead of us." On another occasion, it was mentioned, "You can get a rough idea of where he lives based on your own ethnicity." A week after her donation she was informed the regulations in the recipient's country would never allow them to know each other's identity. However, six months after donation day she would be allowed to know if he survived. Curiously, she may then write to him but may not reveal any personal information about herself, including age, gender and location. Michelle is okay with this.

She expressed, "I wish that I could meet my recipient one day and pray his country's regulations will change to allow this. We are tied for life now, and since I will probably never have children of my own, he is the only living being who has my blood as part of the reason that he is alive. It is hard for me to not know him, but knowing him is not why I donated. If this is how it has to be, then I can live with that. I am not responsible for the outcome."

Michelle wants to share her experiences "so that others might see that there is nothing to fear in this incredible process. It isn't a path that everyone is called to walk. We are each called on our own individual journey. If someone were inspired to walk it too, I hope they'll see that it is life-altering, but in the best possible way."

The guiding principles that saw her through periods of fear or doubt were: "God had not told me to come here to cure this young man of cancer. He asked me to sign up. He asked me to show up. He asked me to give with as much love as I am capable and then maybe a little bit more. And as in everything else in life, really, He is going to do the rest."

The Future

A major goal of hematopoietic stem cell transplantation (HSCT) research is to eliminate graft-versus-host disease (GVHD). A study published in October 2012 showed patients who received HSCs harvested from an unrelated donor's bone marrow were significantly less likely to develop GVHD than those who received HSCs from a donor's peripheral blood. Graft failure was more common among recipients of bone marrow, but chronic GVHD was more common among recipients of peripheral blood stem cell grafts. Whether the more invasive procedure of donating bone marrow results in fewer potential donors stepping up to the plate is unknown.

In March 2013, scientists at Weill Cornell Medical College and the Memorial-Sloan Kettering Cancer Center created a protein to expand the number of adult HSCs after being removed from the marrow of a donor. The protein keeps the expanded HSCs in a stem cell like state, preventing them from differentiating into specialized blood cells before they are transplanted into the recipient's bone marrow. Differentiating means developing or maturing into different types of adult blood cells. This ability opens up new possibilities that could not otherwise be accomplished with current technology.

With this method, not as many stem cells need to be harvested from donors. Adult stem cells could be frozen and stored for future expansion and usage. The cells can be categorized before being frozen and banked so all their HLA types will be known beforehand. Then, when a patient needs a hematopoietic stem cell transplant, cells that match can be quickly identified, expanded and used on a timely basis. The opportunity is also afforded for persons to store their own HSCs for their own potential use or for a family member.

New discoveries like this will certainly help to facilitate more donors because the process is less invasive and the results can be stored for an extended period of time. These medical advances are integral to facilitating an increasing numbers of successful transplantations and as a result, saving more lives. As medical science continues to evolve and transplantation education is further disseminated to the public, Dr. Don Thomas' dedication and unflagging work ethic will ultimately result in touching the lives of donors and recipients alike.

Some final thoughts: There are two figures on the Nobel medal for physiology or medicine. Both are women. One is the Genius of Medicine, who holds an open book in her lap, collecting water pouring out from a rock to quench the thirst of a sick girl. The name of the laureate is engraved on the plate below the figures. The inscription reads: "Inventas vitam juvat excoluisse per artes." These Latin words are taken from Virgil's Aeneid, the sixth song, verse 663. Loosely translated, it means: "They who bettered life on Earth by new-found mastery."

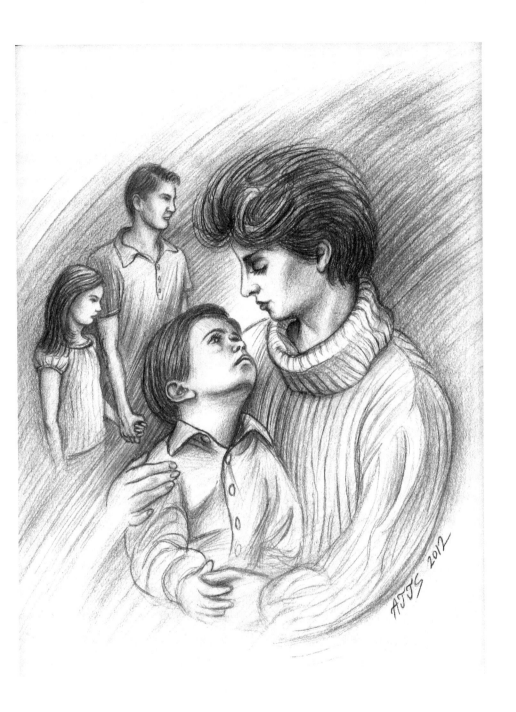

Jehovah's Witnesses

Although the setting was perfect, it was to be our first and last date, but I didn't know that. It was a Saturday night in early June 1970, and we were each sipping a Mai Tai as we gazed through the picture window of the Polynesia Restaurant on Pier 51 in Seattle. The sun was just setting over the Olympic mountain range. We had not ordered dinner when my beeper chirped, and I looked down to see the telephone number of Seattle's county hospital, Harborview. From a nearby public phone, I was patched through to the chief resident in pediatrics. He requested an immediate consultation for a 6-year-old boy seriously ill with diphtheria and a bleeding disorder the resident believed was caused by the diphtheria.

As I returned to the table, I wondered how this child could have diphtheria. Wasn't that disease eradicated in this country through immunization? Although I had never seen a case of diphtheria, I tried to recall what I had read about it and what had been covered in my infectious disease and pediatrics classes. My last thought before placing enough cash on the table to cover the cost of the drinks and a generous tip was: what is the connection between diphtheria and the child's bleeding disorder? Considering this question was the reason the resident called me, I had better come up with an answer and figure out what to do about it.

I explained the situation to my date. As we hurriedly left the restaurant, our waitress asked, with a concerned look, if there was something wrong with the service. I quickly assured her the service was fine, but I had an emergency call. She was visibly relieved.

Being preoccupied about what I would encounter with the patient, it was only when I arrived at the hospital did I realize I had a date sitting next to me in the car. I asked her if she would mind waiting in the hematology office while I performed the consultation. She looked a bit dumbfounded but realized there were really no other options. After I stashed her in an office at the end of a dark, isolated corridor on the second floor, I raced up to the third floor to room 305.

An intern and the chief resident in pediatrics stood at the young patient's bed side. The chief resident was adjusting the dials on a ventilator machine connected to a clear plastic tube placed down the child's throat into his trachea (windpipe). The resident muttered, "I don't understand why this kid requires so much PEEP."

PEEP means positive end-expiratory pressure. It is the pressure above atmospheric pressure required for the mechanical ventilator to push oxygen through the endotracheal tube and into the lungs of a patient who is oxygen-starved, allowing the patient to exhale through the tube. The higher the PEEP setting, the greater the obstruction to airflow in the patient's lungs the ventilator has to overcome.

The resident continued, "The endotracheal tube is in good position past the membrane, so why should there still be an obstruction?"

The membrane he referred to consists of a collection of bacteria that cause diphtheria, dead cells from the lining of the nose and throat, clotted plasma, pus and red blood cells. The membrane coats the nose and throat and develops as a result of a toxin released by the bacteria. It first appears as a thick white coating, which becomes dirty gray with patches of green or black as the disease progresses. It can choke off breathing by obstructing air flow into the lungs. The chief resident could not explain why increased pressure had to be applied to get the oxygenated air into the lungs if the tube was past the obstructing membrane.

One possible reason for the high pressure might have been that, in children, the membrane could extend into the trachea and smaller airways (known as bronchi), causing swelling of the tissues. If untreated, the swelling of the trachea and bronchi could reduce and eventually block air flow, resulting in oxygen deprivation and suffocation.

Every time the machine allowed the boy to exhale through the tube—especially when he coughed—a visible gush of bright red blood would surge into the endotracheal tube. Purplish discolorations of his skin appeared at all the sites where needles had been inserted to draw blood samples and where intravenous fluids and medications entered his veins. The boy also had purple blotches beneath the skin around his eyes, pinpoint red spots of blood on his cheeks, and a swollen neck.

Preliminary laboratory tests revealed low levels of hemoglobin (the substance that transports oxygen in the blood) and platelets (the blood cells that protect us from bleeding and bruising). Screening tests showed the blood took an abnormally long time to clot. We suspected the boy was experiencing disseminated intravascular coagulation (DIC). In DIC, problems with the clotting mechanism result in depletion of the coagulation factors necessary for a good, strong blood clot to form, causing the patient to have uncontrolled bleeding.

I said, "The laboratory data certainly support DIC. We have to transfuse him with a unit of fresh whole blood, not banked blood, to supply him with the red blood cells, platelets and coagulation factors that are depleted. What blood group and Rh type is he?"

"A-positive," the resident replied.

"Great," I exclaimed, "I'm A-positive too. We can draw a unit of my blood for a cross-match and transfuse him right away."

"Not so fast," the chief resident said. "This is a Jehovah's Witness child. We have initiated proceedings to have him made a ward of the court. The circuit court judge will be here at 6 a.m. in the board room. The boy's father has refused to allow us to transfuse him, saying that it's contrary to his religious beliefs to do so. Although he has not allowed his son to receive any immunizations in the past, he has allowed us to use the antitoxin, which we've already administered, and we've also started him on erythromycin. But the father is adamant about the blood. We have to document that his son has DIC and that there is a need for the transfusion. Every "i" has to be dotted and every "t" has to be crossed before we meet with the judge. On weekends, the coagulation technologist from University Hospital is on call for Harborview, but we've been unable to reach her. Can you help us out here?"

I had what I thought was the perfect solution. Having spent nine months at Children's Hospital of Seattle in the pediatric hematology/oncology department as part of my fellowship training, I knew the Children's coagulation technologist, Mary Willeman, was on call 24/7. Her life was devoted to children with bleeding disorders. I called the chief of pediatric hematology/oncology at Children's, Dr. Jack Hartmann, and obtained his permission to call in Mary to perform the necessary tests in her lab.

Then Dr. Hartmann asked a question that made me feel intimidated. "Why wasn't the pediatric hematologist at Harborview or his fellow asked to see that boy?"

"I didn't know they had a pediatric fellowship program here," I replied.

Dr. Hartmann exclaimed, "Sure, the chairman of the pediatrics department at Harborview is a hematologist."

I responded, "Maybe the chief resident knew me from my rotations through Children's and assumed that I was a pediatric hematology fellow rather than an adult hematology fellow. I don't know, but the ball is now in my court since the judge will be here in the morning." With tubes of the boy's blood in hand, I retrieved my date from the office where she had sat forlornly for at least an hour, and I drove with her across town to Children's Hospital. I dropped off the specimens of blood to Mary, who was already in her lab. Then I dropped off my date, who lived near the hospital. Before I could get out of the car to open her door (a mostly forgotten courtesy these days), she literally jumped out of the car.

I said, "I'll call you tomorrow and tell you how everything worked out."

She turned her head and with a cold stare replied, "Don't bother," as she bounded up the stairs to her home.

Although I felt somewhat dejected, I realized there could never be any future in a relationship with someone who obviously could not contend with the life of a doctor, especially when my duties involved a critically ill child.

I returned to Mary's lab at Children's Hospital, where I prepared and stained some blood from the child. The blood showed fragmentation of his red blood cells and a low number of platelets, confirming the destructive mechanism associated with DIC that was contributing to his anemia. With these observations written on a lab slip and with the rest of the lab reports documenting the DIC process, I returned to Harborview. It was about midnight. During the six hours before the judge's arrival, the chief resident filled me in on the rest of the story.

Not only was this case a medical and religious disaster, it was a societal and political hot potato as well. The boy's family was from Marysville, Washington, a strawberry-farming community 35 miles north of Seattle. Just to the west of Marysville is the Tulalip Indian Reservation. In 1969, a federal judge issued an order for mandatory busing of Native American children from that reservation into the Marysville school system. Historically, the health care of reservation Indians was administered by the United States Public Health System (USPHS) Bureau of Indian Affairs. In 1955, responsibility for Native American health care was transferred to the newly created Indian Health Service, which reported to the surgeon general but was staffed by USPHS officers. It appeared that, somehow, a number of children on the reservation had not received their usual course of childhood vaccinations, including that for diphtheria. These children apparently became infected with diphtheria and introduced it to the Marysville children.

You typically get diphtheria by breathing in the bacteria after an infected person has coughed or sneezed. You can also get it from contact with discharges from an infected person's mouth, nose, throat or skin. In this case, the only Marysville children who became infected were members of a Jehovah's Witness family who had purposively not been vaccinated because the parents considered the vaccine to be a blood product. The boy's mother and older sister were also hospitalized in Harborview with diphtheria. The father, who had not contracted the disease, informed us that while doing noncombat-related public service as a conscientious objector in an Army-base hospital during the Vietnam era, he suffered a leg fracture. The doctors considered the wound to be potentially contaminated and gave the father—to his subsequent knowledge—the combination diphtheria-tetanus toxoid vaccine. This vaccine later apparently protected him from the disease contracted by his wife and children.

Vaccinations were banned by Jehovah's Witnesses from 1921 to 1952. The policy seems to have changed during the 1940s. Of approximately 4,300 Witnesses who were in prison as conscientious objectors during WWII, only a small minority who were concentrated in one prison refused to submit to vaccination, compulsory for all inmates. In December 1952, a neutral posture was assumed, stating in their official publication, the Watchtower, "it would be up to the Bible-trained conscience of the individual as to whether (a member of their faith) would accept vaccinations for himself and his family."

Aside from Christian Scientists, Jehovah's Witnesses are not the only group who has expressed a religious objection to vaccination. Some vaccines contain trypsin and/or gelatin of pork origin which is objectionable to Jews and Muslims. Some are manufactured using cell lines derived from a human fetus that has been aborted, which is objectionable to Catholics and other prolife Christians. However, Jewish, Islamic and Catholic religious leaders have issued statements indicating support for the use of these vaccines if alternatives are not available.

At 6 Sunday morning, I entered the board room. At the near end of the table sat the judge, court recorder and the child's father. On the left sat a distinguished-looking older physician, who later identified himself as the chairman of the pediatrics department, and a younger physician, who appeared to be about my age and was later identified as the pediatric hematology fellow. Both doctors wore long white lab coats. Sitting directly across from the judge at the far end of the table were the chief resident in pediatrics and his intern. I sat alone on the right side of the table, close to the child's father. The judge began the proceedings by explaining the reasons for the hearing, as the court stenographer pecked away at her instrument, recording every word. The judge then asked that each doctor in the room describe the educational background and training that qualified him to render an opinion as to the necessity of a blood transfusion in the treatment of the child. I was the last physician to speak and merely echoed what the others had said about the indication for the transfusion.

Next, the judge gave the boy's father the opportunity to state his objection to treatment of his son with blood. The father spoke softly but with conviction. My first reaction was that he was unusually articulate for a man identified as a strawberry farmer. He proceeded to explain, "I and my family are Jehovah's Witnesses. I am the head of my household and am responsible for the spiritual, financial and moral support of my family. I have raised my children to be Jehovah's Witnesses. My understanding of the Bible, which guides my life, tells me that we must not take blood into our body. For this reason, I cannot and will not accept a blood transfusion for my son. I realize that he is in grave danger of death. But to violate my religious beliefs by allowing you to transfuse my son with blood would offend my God, Jehovah, at a time when I need Him most."

In response to the father's sincere plea, my thoughts were, "Oh my God! I don't want any part in transfusing this child. I am sorry that I volunteered the use of my blood. I will never again participate in the transfusion of blood or any blood product that violates the conscience of Jehovah's Witnesses or their children. I want out of this!"

Immediately after the father spoke, the judge sternly proclaimed, "With the authority vested in me by the county of King in the city of Seattle, I hereby declare [the patient to be] a ward of the court, and in the medical judgment of his physicians, his health requires a blood transfusion, which I duly authorize." He then pounded his gavel three times. On the third bang of the gavel, the PA system announced, "Code Blue, Code Blue, room 305." All the doctors jumped up from the table and ran up two flights of stairs to what we all knew was the child's fate in room 305—cardiac arrest. Attempts at resuscitation were futile.

We all gathered in a nearby lounge area with the boy's father. The room had a small adjoining glass-enclosed anteroom filled with people whom I assumed were family members. Each doctor gave his condolences to the child's father. The longest conversation was with the chief resident. I was the last to approach the father. I told him, "I am very sorry about your loss. A decision has been made by a power greater than the court. I want you to know that I was moved by your plea to not transfuse your son by explaining why it would be a violation of your religious beliefs. I now believe that you have every right to make that decision for your children. Rest assured, I will never participate in this type of court proceeding again. I will respect the right of conscience of the members of your faith to refuse blood for themselves and their children." He thanked me and returned to the anteroom.

The chief resident approached me and said, "He has refused an autopsy. You seem to have some rapport with him. Ask him for permission to do a post-mortem on his son."

"Why do you want it?"

"I still don't know why the boy required so much PEEP, and I don't know if raising it did more harm than good. I'm hoping that an autopsy will tell us. Besides, we really don't know much about diphtheria. Since the advent of immunization for diphtheria, none of us, including the chairman of the department, have ever seen a case. I'm hoping that what we learn from a post-mortem examination will be useful in treating the wife and daughter in the event that their conditions deteriorate."

That sounded reasonable to me, so I asked the father to step out of the anteroom and inquired whether the performance of an autopsy on his son was against his religious beliefs. He asked why the autopsy was being requested, and I gave him the answer I had received from the chief resident. The father indicated he would confer with the elders of his congregation in the anteroom.

I learned that all congregations of Jehovah's Witnesses have a body of elders to provide needed spiritual and emotional support to each member. The members feel the elders know best the convictions of their faith and can assist families and the medical community to resolve problems that arise pertaining to the use of blood. More recently, Jehovah's Witnesses have established hospital liaison committees of specially trained elders in all major cities to facilitate communication between doctors and Witness patients. These committees help support Witness families and attending physicians by assisting with doctor or hospital referrals, locating medical teams experienced in non-blood management techniques, facilitating doctor to doctor consultations and providing medical information from a large reference library. Their resources include case specific research and medical articles about emergency management. When the boy's father returned from consulting the elders, he informed us there was no biblical-based proscription against a post-mortem examination. Thus, he would grant permission for the autopsy with two conditions. The first condition was that I was to attend it, and the second was I would report to him whatever findings might help in the care of his wife and daughter. I agreed.

The autopsy not only answered the chief resident's question about the required PEEP, but it provided information immediately useful in the treatment of the wife and daughter, as well as other patients with diphtheria. Not unexpectedly, the membrane that began developing in the child's throat had extended into the windpipe and first branches of airways in the lungs—the primary bronchi. However, beyond the membrane, there was a clear swelling of the lining of the next division of the airways—the secondary bronchi— deeper in the lungs. This swelling was so intense it glistened. Air could pass only through a needle-thin channel. This is why the PEEP had to be set so high to push the air through the almost completely blocked smaller air passages well beyond the membrane.

Armed with this information, we decided to administer cortisone-like steroids—designed to shrink the swelling in the lining of the airways—to the wife and daughter. We also administered diuretics to reduce the water content of the air passages. I reported our findings and changes in strategy to the father as he prayed at the bedside of his daughter. He gave me a simple but sincere thank you.

Jehovah's Witnesses are a worldwide Christian society of people who actively bear witness regarding Jehovah God and His purposes affecting mankind. They base their beliefs solely on the Bible. The modern-day history of Jehovah's Witnesses began with the forming of a Bible study group in Allegheny, Pennsylvania, near Pittsburgh, in 1872 by the American clergyman Charles Taze

Russell. At first, they were known only as Bible Students, but in 1931 they adopted the Scriptural name, Jehovah's Witnesses (Isaiah 43:10-12). Their beliefs and practices are not new, but rather a restoration of first-century Christianity. Jesus said He would have on Earth a "faithful and discreet slave" (his anointed followers viewed as a group), through which he would provide spiritual food to those making up the household of faith (Matthew 24:45-47). Jehovah's Witnesses recognize that arrangement. As was true of first-century Christians, they look to the governing body of that "faithful and discrete slave" class to resolve difficult questions—not on the basis of human wisdom, but by drawing on their knowledge of the Bible, on God's dealings with His servants, and on help from God's spirit, for which they earnestly pray (Acts 15:1-29; 16:4-5). Although there are many branch locations, the world headquarters of Jehovah's Witnesses, the Watchtower Bible and Tract Society, is in Brooklyn, New York. In 2012, there were 1,203,552 Jehovah's Witnesses in the United States, including almost 30,000 in the Detroit metropolitan area.

Jehovah's Witnesses actively seek the highest quality of modern, scientific medical care for themselves and their families. They do not subscribe to faith healing. However, they do object to blood transfusions. They avail themselves of health insurance plans that provide the utmost degree of flexibility in choosing physicians who respect their religious and medical reasons for this objection, as well as hospitals in which this objection is honored. The antitransfusion position taken by the Witnesses is a religious one, based on their understanding of the Bible, regardless of medical risk factors. They make a concerted effort to identify health care personnel who will not threaten or cajole them regarding this issue and who avoid deceit, manipulation, arrogance and hardline authoritarianism. They especially eschew attempts to have them sign waivers to accept blood transfusions. Such waivers are sometimes asked of patients scheduled to undergo elective surgical procedures, even in the absence of life-threatening situations and in cases in which the need for transfusions may never arise.

Medical alternatives to blood transfusions are vigorously pursued by Jehovah's Witnesses, who are the best-educated consumers of bloodless medicine and surgery techniques. There are a variety of such techniques, all designed to avoid the need for blood transfusions. For example, fluids called crystalloids and colloids can be used to maintain fluid volume in blood vessels when the patient loses blood, and certain biological stimulants of red blood cells, white blood cells and platelets (the blood elements that protect us from bleeding and bruising) can be used to increase the production of these blood components from the patient's own bone marrow. Because of misunderstandings regarding their beliefs and what they will or will not accept in medical care, the Watchtower Society has taken a proactive and assertive role in the education of physicians and hospital personnel regarding alternatives to blood. More than 1,700 hospital liaison committees have been established by Jehovah's Witnesses to provide a spiritual support system for their members and a network to provide authoritative information regarding clinical strategies to avoid blood transfusion and facilitate access to health care for patients who are Jehovah's Witnesses. I have participated on several occasions in medical and surgical conferences sponsored by hospital liaison committees and given presentations about my experiences in the medical care of Jehovah' Witnesses.

Some physicians may assume defensive postures when given the admittedly difficult challenge of identifying and employing non-blood alternatives to conventional treatments. Furthermore, some doctors may totally abrogate their roles in patient care by referring Witnesses to other physicians who will honor their religious-based refusal of blood.

Jehovah's Witnesses are a deeply religious people who believe blood transfusions are forbidden by commands contained in the Bible. Their preferred version of the Bible is the New World Translation of the Holy Scriptures, translated from the original scriptural languages by the New World Bible Translation Committee (as revised in 2013) and published by the Watchtower Society. In the Bible, a command given to Noah and his family after The Flood, found in Genesis 9:3, 4, is translated from the original Hebrew and Aramaic scriptures:

"Every moving animal that is alive may serve as food for you. As in the case of green vegetation, I do give it all to you. Only flesh with its life—its blood—you must not eat."

Found in Leviticus 17:13, 14, is this command to the nation of Israel as delivered through Moses:

"If one of the Israelites or some foreigner who is residing in your midst is hunting and catches a wild animal or a bird that may be eaten, he must pour its blood out and cover it with dust. For the life of every sort of flesh is its blood, because the life is in it. Consequently, I said to the Israelites: "You must not eat the blood of any sort of flesh, because the life of every sort of flesh is its blood. Anyone eating it will be cut off."

It is this passage that is the basis for kosher dietary law requiring exsanguination of an animal before consumption of its flesh

In the New Testament, the proscription against blood is found in Acts of the Apostles 15:28, 29:

"For the holy spirit and we ourselves have favored adding no further burden to you, except those necessary things, to keep abstaining from things sacrificed to idols, from blood, from what is strangled and from sexual immorality. If you carefully keep yourselves from these things, you will prosper. Good health to you!"
Beginning in 1992, the Watchtower Society published a handbook titled Family Care and Medical Management for Jehovah's Witnesses, which is continually updated and is made available to physicians, judges, social workers and other professionals who may become involved in health care decisions involving children of

Jehovah's Witnesses. The handbook states that the three biblical references mentioned above form the basis for the Jehovah's Witness belief that, "Taking blood into one's body through mouth or veins violates God's laws." Obviously, these verses of the Bible are not written in medical terminology. Nevertheless, the Watchtower Society, the governing body of the Jehovah's Witness faith, decided in 1945 that taking blood into one's body is nourishment. The issue arose when the transfusion of blood emerged as common practice during the years of World War II. The elders reasoned that although blood cannot be eaten as nourishment, intravenous blood is given in much the same way as parenteral nutrition (that is, through the veins); thus, giving blood is equivalent to nourishment. With this association made, Witnesses believe the three cited biblical passages, in addition to several others, rule out transfusion of whole blood, plasma, red blood cells, white blood cells and platelets.

When asked if a blood transfusion is really the same as eating blood, the response found in the 2009 edition of "Reasoning from the Scripture" published by the Watchtower Bible and Tract Society is:

"In a hospital, when a patient cannot eat through his mouth, he is fed intravenously. Now, would a person who never put blood in his mouth but who accepted blood by transfusion really be obeying the command to 'keep abstaining from...blood' (Acts 15:29)? To use a comparison, consider a man who is told by the doctor that he must abstain from alcohol. Would he be obedient if he quit drinking alcohol but had it put directly into his veins? Since the Bible shows that it is necessary to please God and requires abstinence from blood, when seeking medical care for ourselves and our children, we ask that the physician use alternatives to blood since keeping God's approval and having a good conscience are paramount to us. We Witness parents believe God's promise that those who are obedient to Him have the hope of everlasting life on our earth restored to a paradise. We want this inheritance for our children as well. We have no desire to martyr ourselves or our children for the sake of our religion. We believe that we have an obligation to God to safeguard our children's health based on such scriptures as 1 Timothy 5:8—certainly if anyone does not provide for those who are his own, and especially for those who are members of his household, he has disowned the faith and is worse than a person without faith."

For Jehovah's Witnesses, abstaining from blood is a very serious matter. The same Bible passage directing Christians to abstain from blood (Acts 15:28, 29) also directs them to abstain from idolatry and sexual immorality. Therefore, Witnesses view the violation of God's word on blood to be as severe a wrong as engaging in false worship or sexual immorality. They consistently declare that they consider the forcible, nonconsensual administration of blood to be morally equivalent to rape.

To willingly accept blood for themselves or their children carries serious psychological and social implications for Witnesses, including the risk of being cut off from their broad community of friends and family. This action is based on the previously noted passage from Leviticus 17:14; "*You must not eat the blood of any sort of flesh, because the life of every sort of flesh is its blood. Anyone eating it will be cut off.*"

In the past, if this weakness of faith did not respond to spiritual assistance, the practice of disfellowshipping was applied to all unrepentant Witnesses who accepted blood transfusions. However, at present, the act of willfully accepting a transfusion, itself, dissociates a Witness spiritually from the body of the faith.

A Witness' religious understanding does not absolutely prohibit the medical use of blood components, such as the albumin, immune globulins and factor concentrates used in the treatment of patients with hemophilia and related bleeding disorders. The same flexibility applies to diagnostic and therapeutic procedures that involve extracting a small amount of a patient's blood, labeling it with a radioactive substance, and then reinjecting it into the patient. The Witness position is that each Witness must individually decide, as a matter of conscience, whether he or she will accept certain blood fractions and related procedures.

Some Witness patients will allow the use of a heart-lung machine or a hemodialysis machine, provided the pump is primed with non-blood fluids and their blood is not stored in the process. Also acceptable to many Jehovah's Witnesses is autotransfusion, in which the patient's blood is collected in a closed circuit linked to the patient's circulatory system, then reintroduced into the patient without interim storage. They do not accept preoperative collection and storage of blood for later transfusion.

During certain surgical procedures, some blood may be diverted from the patient's body in a process call hemodilution. This blood-conservation technique is a type of autotransfusion that entails the removal of one to three units of blood (450-500 milliliters constitutes one unit) from a patient, either immediately before or shortly after the induction of anesthesia. A normal volume of circulating fluids is maintained by the addition of crystalloids and colloids, the non-blood fluids previously discussed. The blood is prevented from clotting and can be maintained at room temperature for as long as eight hours in a closed circuit outside the patient's body. This blood is recirculated into the patient as needed during or after the surgical procedure. This technique is best suited to use with healthy, young adults who have a normal number of red blood cells and who are expected to lose more than two units of blood during the procedure.

Similarly, another type of autotransfusion is a procedure called intraoperative blood salvage (IBS), when blood that flows into a surgical wound is suctioned and filtered so that the patient's own red blood cells can be returned to the individual. This blood-conservation technique is considered acceptable by some Jehovah's Witnesses provided their blood does not leave their extended circulatory system. As with the hemodilution technique, the equipment must be arranged in a closed circuit constantly linked to the patient's circulatory system. But the IBS technique is unique among transfusion methods because of its capacity to rapidly provide immense quantities of autologous blood (blood for which the donor and recipient are the same person). It can be used throughout a surgical procedure to replace blood in proportion to the volume lost.

Each individual Jehovah's Witness faced with making a decision regarding any of these medical procedures is urged to carefully and prayerfully weigh matters and then decide conscientiously what to do before God. Most physicians respect such decisions from Jehovah's Witness adults capable of giving informed consent to refuse any form of medical or surgical treatment for themselves. Yet, there are physicians whose moral or ethical codes of conduct do not accept this right of refusal regarding blood transfusions for competent adult patients in critical condition whose lives, in their judgment, might be saved with transfusions. Such a physician should refer the patient to another physician, one who does respect the religious beliefs of the patient and who has experience with bloodless medicine. Almost universally, physicians face ethical or moral problems when parents or guardians refuse blood transfusions for their young children or their mentally challenged adult children. Despite the provision of an identity card that identifies the child as one of Jehovah's Witnesses who does not accept a blood transfusion, when there is an actual or potential need for administration of blood or blood products to an immature Witness patient, the medical personnel and hospital administration typically try to pressure the parents to grant permission to transfuse their child.

If the application of such pressure is unsuccessful, a petition for medical treatment is typically filed with a circuit court judge alleging the parents are failing to provide adequate medical care (cf MCL712A.2(b)((1) or that the child's health requires it (cf MCL

722.634). The court is typically petitioned to have the child declared a temporary ward of the court. With 1.2 million Jehovah's Witnesses in the United States, the blood transfusion issue places a large number of health care providers in conflict with Jehovah's Witnesses. One researcher has estimated the annual rate of Jehovah's Witness minors who require a blood transfusion is one case for every 1,000 Jehovah's Witnesses in the U.S. population. That estimate would mean there are more than 1,200 cases each year in the United States in which a hospital seeks a court order to administer what is deemed to be medically necessary blood transfusions over parental objections. In August 2011, the State's Attorney for Broward County, Florida, reported his office handled 12 cases in the previous three years in which Jehovah's Witness parents refused life-saving blood transfusions for their minor children.

When the court takes custody of a child, it is saying a particular decision by the parents is not in the best interest of the child. The judge may then appoint a temporary guardian who makes medical decisions for the child over the parents' objections. It is largely held that in the event of an immediate life-threatening situation that requires any medical intervention, including blood transfusion, that under the physician's right of emergency power, a court order is not needed to transfuse a minor because that right lies with the physician himself.

Organ Transplants

No biblical command specifically forbids a Jehovah's Witness from accepting an organ transplant such as heart, kidney, liver, lung or pancreas. Some Witnesses will accept a bone marrow transplant.

Bone marrow is the soft, spongy tissue inside some of the larger bones of the body. This marrow produces all the cells found in the blood, including red blood cells, white blood cells of several types, and platelets. All these cells develop from precursor cells in the bone marrow called hematopoietic stem cells. Most of these stem cells stay in the marrow until they transform into the various blood cells, which are then released into the blood stream. Many patients with cancer are given high doses of chemotherapy or radiation intended to kill the abnormal, cancer cells in their bodies. Unfortunately, these treatments also destroy the normal cells developing in the bone marrow, including the stem cells. After such treatment, the patient is given a new supply of healthy hematopoietic stem cells previously been harvested from his or her body or from a donor. These stem cells can be derived from the bone marrow (in a bone marrow transplant), from the bloodstream (in a peripheral blood stem cell transplant), or from the umbilical cord blood of a healthy newborn (in an umbilical cord blood transplant). In this way, the blood cell production process can be reestablished in the marrow of a patient.

For bone marrow transplantation, the marrow is typically removed, under anesthesia, from the pelvis of the patient or from that of a donor before chemotherapy or radiation and then frozen for storage and later use. The donor is usually a brother or sister of the patient. The donor may also be an unrelated person with a matched genetic profile of what are known as histocompatibility locus antigens or HLA type compatible with the recipient's tissues. After the chemotherapy or radiation is completed, the harvested stem cells are thawed and injected into the patient through a vein, and they take up residence in their natural habitat of the bone marrow.

The scriptural basis for a Jehovah's Witness to accept a bone marrow transplant is that Isaiah spoke of eating bone marrow (Isaiah 25:6), *"And Jehovah of armies will certainly make for all the peoples, in this mountain, a banquet of well-oiled dishes, a banquet of [wine kept on] the dregs, of well-oiled dishes filled with marrow, of [wine kept on] the dregs, filtered."*

Quoting again from the 2009 version of "Reasoning from the Scripture" published by the Watchtower Society of New York: "If one were to say to a Jehovah's Witness, 'Since the Bible states clearly that God's servants must abstain from blood. (Acts 15:28, 29; Deuteronomy 12:15, 16) and, since red cells originate in the red bone marrow,' do the Scriptures class marrow with blood?"

They would respond: "No. In fact, animal marrow is spoken of like any other flesh that could be eaten. Isaiah 25:6 says God will prepare for his people a banquet that includes 'well-oiled dishes filled with marrow'. Normal slaughtering and drainage procedures never drain all blood cells from the marrow. Yet once a carcass is drained, then any of the tissue may be eaten, including the marrow. Of course, marrow used in human marrow transplants is from live donors, and the withdrawn marrow may have some blood in it. Hence the Christian would have to resolve for himself whether to him the bone marrow graft would amount to simple flesh or would be unbled tissue. Additionally, since a marrow graft is a form of transplant, the Scriptural aspects of human organ transplants should be considered."

Since virtually all marrow transplant recipients will require platelet and red blood cell transfusions, Jehovah's Witnesses would have to consider what additional issues they would have to face if they submitted to a marrow transplant.

Small numbers of hematopoietic stem cells can also be found in the circulating blood. Collecting these peripheral blood stem cells is similar to the process used for harvesting blood platelets. An apparatus called an apheresis device, or cell separator, is used to remove hematopoietic stem cells from blood by a filtration process. The patient receiving the cells is most commonly treated with a growth factor, called granulocyte colony-stimulating factor, to stimulate production of the cells so there will be a sufficient number of them in the blood. If not viewed as one of the primary components of blood, collecting, freezing and storage of peripheral blood stem cells is not a prohibitive issue for Witnesses. Though a personal decision has to be made, the Bible's comments about blood and marrow should help the individual to decide. The decision on this matter is based on their Bible-trained conscience, not merely subjectivity.

Using the patient's own bone marrow or peripheral blood stem cells is called an autologous transplantation. Using a donor's bone marrow or peripheral blood stem cells is called an allogeneic transplantation. The donors of an allogeneic transplantation may be related or unrelated. Siblings who share the same parents are typically the only family members who are tested as potential donors because they have a one in four chance of being sufficiently HLA compatible to serve as a suitable donor. In general, parents, children and relatives are not suitable donors since they do not share the same parents. A notable exception, as mentioned in the chapters on twins and bone marrow transplantation, is the rare instance when identical twins marry identical twins. All their children would be genetic siblings as opposed to cousins. Those without siblings or if HLA testing does not reveal a match, a matched unrelated donor may be identified using transplant registries throughout the world.

Over the past ten years, peripheral blood stem cells derived from circulating blood have equaled bone marrow as a source for stem cells used in transplantation. But bone marrow transplants now account for only 24 percent of the grafts from unrelated adult donors for patients with blood cancers. This is due to several factors outlined in the chapter on bone marrow transplantation.

Graft-versus-host disease (GVHD) is a common complication of either a bone marrow or peripheral blood stem cell transplant in which someone receives the graft from a donor (allogeneic). The graft refers to the transplanted hematopoietic stem cells. The host refers to the patient (recipient). It does not occur when persons receive their own marrow or peripheral blood stem cells (autologous) and very rarely from an identical twin. GVHD occurs when the graft contains viable and functional immune cells (T cells), the recipient is not truly HLA identical, and the recipient is immune compromised and cannot destroy or activate the transplanted T cells. The T cells regard the recipient's body as foreign and begin to attack the host's body cells. This is expressed largely in the skin, digestive tract and liver. The severity of GVHD is less with those who receive closely matched bone marrow or peripheral blood stem cells and worse with increasing age of the host.

Acute GVHD develops within the first 100 days following an allogeneic transplant. It is marked by:

Skin rash, itching and redness

Abdominal pain or cramps, nausea, vomiting and diarrhea

Dry or irritated eyes

Jaundice seen as yellowing of the skin or eyes

Chronic GVHD usually starts beyond 100 days after transplantation and can last a lifetime. Symptoms include:

Dry eyes or vision changes

Dry mouth, white patches inside the mouth and sensitivity to spicy foods

Fatigue, muscle weakness and chronic pain

Skin rash with raised, discolored areas, as well as skin tightening or thickening

Shortness of breath

Vaginal dryness

Weight loss

Previous studies of matched sibling donors have shown that peripheral blood stem cells accelerate engraftment (successful transplantation) but increase the risk of acute and chronic graft-versus-host disease compared with transplantation of bone marrow.

A study, published in October 2012, compared stem cells obtained from peripheral blood with bone marrow grafts in patients undergoing matched but unrelated donor transplantation. All the patients were younger than 65 years and suffered from those blood cancers that account for 75 percent of the unrelated-donor transplantations in the U.S.—acute leukemia, myelodysplasia, chronic myeloid or myelomonocytic leukemia or myelofibrosis. The study concluded that rates of survival, relapse and acute graft-versus-host disease are similar with peripheral blood stem cell and bone marrow grafts. However, there were significant differences. Engraftment was quicker and failure to engraft was lower with peripheral blood progenitor cells (3 percent versus 9 percent) but the rate of chronic graft-versus-host is lower with a bone marrow graft at two years post-transplant (41percent versus 53 percent). This might be expected since peripheral blood contains at least twice as many T cells as bone marrow.

In an allogeneic transplant, the donor's immune system—generated from the transplanted hematopoietic stem cells—recognize your cells, including leukemic cells, as foreign and rejects them. This beneficial reaction is called graft versus leukemia effect. The immune response caused by the transplanted cells improves the overall effectiveness of the treatment. It is a reality that Jehovah's Witnesses would receive reduced intensity anti-leukemic chemotherapy (mini-transplantation as explained in the chapter on bone marrow transplantation) in an attempt to avoid lethal bone marrow depression of normal blood cell production while attempting to eradicate their leukemic cells. Patients who have reduced intensity chemotherapy have a higher risk of graft failure and should use peripheral blood transplants because of higher engraftment rates. It is hoped that with this mini transplant, the graft versus leukemia effect of the same T cells that contribute to graft-versus-host disease will eradicate any remaining leukemia cells in the host. This is a very real and important consideration for Jehovah's Witnesses considering a bone marrow versus peripheral blood stem cell transplantation since theologically they tend to favor the former.

The Physician's Challenge

Jehovah's Witnesses pose a dilemma and challenge for the physician dedicated to preserving life and health by employing all the techniques at his or her disposal. The ethical principles of autonomy and beneficence come into conflict when a physician believes a blood transfusion is in the best interest of the patient, but the patient refuses this procedure. Physicians have a responsibility to promote the patient's well-being, especially physical health, and they have a moral obligation to always act in their patient's best interest. To not give a blood transfusion in a life-threatening situation may violate a physician's personal, moral, ethical, cultural or religious convictions.

Many physicians of my vintage have practiced with a philosophy of paternalism and beneficence. Their rationale for giving blood transfusions, despite the protestations of a patient or the parents of a patient, is a feeling of moral obligation. To do otherwise would be a breach of their medical ethics. In such circumstances, the physician disagrees with the patient's value system, which is viewed as preventing the physician from doing what he or she believes is right and possibly saving a life. The physician may find it unacceptable to watch someone die when that individual's life could be saved by a relatively simple procedure.

Today's younger physicians are taught to respect a patient's autonomy and health care preferences, which—for adults who are capable of informed consent—have been protected in court challenges since 1985. It is, perhaps, no coincidence that hospital programs dedicated to bloodless medicine, including multiple blood-conservation methods, debuted soon after these court challenges began.

The State

Although the state has an interest in the preservation of life, that interest is not absolute. It has been well tested in the courts that individuals have the right to control their own person, and part of that autonomy is the right to make choices pertaining to one's health, including the right to refuse unwanted treatment. Even for competent adult Jehovah's Witnesses, this right had to be defended in the courts until 1985, when an appellate court in Mississippi ended the debate from a legal perspective with a strongly worded statement supporting an individual's right to refuse medical treatment:

"Rights are subject to compromise only when they collide with conflicting rights vested in others...The right of free exercise of religion protects more than mere beliefs...Religiously grounded actions or conduct are often beyond the authority of the state to control."

The court ordered that a "competent and alert adult...shall not be required to submit to or receive a transfusion of blood against her will, notwithstanding any interest the State of Mississippi may claim in this matter."

This statement, which has been supported by subsequent court cases, recognizes that competent adult Jehovah's Witnesses have the legal right to refuse unwanted blood products. This right extends to the issue of whether a competent, pregnant Witness woman's right to refuse medical treatment involving blood transfusions may be overridden by the state's interest in the welfare of her fetus. In 1997, an Illinois appellate court held "that the State may not override a pregnant woman's competent treatment decision, including refusal of recommended invasive medical procedures, to save the life of the viable fetus." This right has not been extended to refusal of medical treatment with blood transfusions for minor children.

Parents Have Rights—Up to a Point

Parents have the responsibility of ensuring the survival of their children, protecting them from injury, and comforting them when necessary. Society recognizes that parents have the authority to rear their children in a manner they consider appropriate for achieving physical and personal development. Many parents believe they alone have authority over, and responsibility for, their children. After all, whose children are they?

In 1979, the chief justice of the Supreme Court of the United States, Warren E. Burger, wrote the majority opinion in Parham v. J.R. that declared:

"...the law's concept of the family rests on the presumption that parents possess what a child lacks in maturity, experience, and capacity for judgment required for making life's difficult decisions... Simply because the decision of the parent [on a medical matter] involves risks does not automatically transfer the power to make that decision from the parents to some agency or officer of the state."

Despite this opinion of the High Court, cases involving blood transfusions for Jehovah's Witness children have invariably been decided in favor of ordering a blood transfusion when a court has been petitioned to do so. Thus, the question remains—do parents have a constitutional right to make the decision to decline a blood transfusion for their child and to exercise their right of conscience? Or does the state have the right to disrupt families over this issue and interfere with parental authority over children? Legal rulings continue to be challenged by attorneys on behalf of Jehovah's Witnesses when their constitutional rights are denied. The courts have decided that although the authority and responsibility for children belong primarily to the parents, society has an interest based on three main principles:

1. The child's interests and those of the state outweigh parental rights to refuse medical treatment.

2. Parental rights do not give parents life and death authority over their children.

3. Parents do not have an absolute right to refuse medical treatment for their children based on their religious beliefs.

Based on these three principles, the rights of Jehovah's Witness parents to refuse blood transfusions for their minor children or infants have been consistently overridden when courts have determined the child's life may be in danger or there is probability of substantial harm or suffering. Jehovah's Witnesses realize parental authority is not absolute. They understand the state has the right to provide treatment believed to be necessary to safeguard a child's life or health.

The courts do not insist on what is standard of care for minors. Otherwise, all parents whose children have crooked teeth would be neglectful if they failed to provide orthodonture or if the physician's choice is chemotherapy but the parents opt for radiation, etc. It is not "no treatment" but "which treatment." The key question that needs to be asked in cases involving children of Witnesses is not whether the parent is refusing standard or indicated care (i.e. homologous blood transfusion therapy) but whether the parent's choice of alternative non-blood management will adequately meet or respond to the child's health care needs. Put another way, is homologous blood indispensably necessary to preserve the child's life or health, or is it merely the standard indicated approach popular among doctors? If it is merely what most doctors would do or what the profession prefers, but the child can be adequately treated with non-blood alternative management sought by the parents, the parents should not be forced to submit to some unnecessary, professionally dictated standard. Certainly, the state has no interest in mandating a rigid standard of medical care for all children if the parents are adequately providing for their children's health care needs.

The traditional presumption of the incompetence of minors has three exceptions: emancipated minors (those who live independently of their parents, who serve in the military, or who are married); minors seeking certain kinds of medical care (such as for contraception, pregnancy, sexually transmitted disease, alcohol and drug abuse, and psychiatric disorders); and mature minors (those deemed able to understand the nature and consequences of medical treatment). The age at which a mature minor is considered capable of giving informed consent varies by state. It is generally held that minors aged 12 and younger do not have the intellectual ability and volition to provide informed, voluntary and rational consent. Most states allow minors aged 13 through 18 to provide consent for medical care.

In 1982, University of Pittsburgh researchers Lois A. Weithorn and Susan B. Campbell studied the competency of children and adolescents to make informed treatment decisions. The researchers concluded that 14-year-olds did not differ from adults according to four standards of competency—evidence of choice, reasonable outcome, rational reasons, and hypothetical dilemmas regarding treatment for different medical conditions. The researchers further found that 9-year-olds appeared less competent than adults according to standards of competency requiring understanding and a rational reasoning process. Yet, according to the standards of evidence of choice and reasonable outcome, these younger minors appeared competent. They comprehended the basics of what was required of them when asked to state a preference regarding a treatment dilemma. Despite poorer understanding and failure to fully consider many elements of disclosed information, the young children tended to express clear and sensible treatment preferences, similar to adults. The investigators concluded that setting the ages of 18 to 21 as the cutoff points below which individuals are perceived to be incompetent to make decisions on their own welfare (which is the law in some states) does not reflect the psychological reality of most adolescents.

If someone were to say to a Jehovah's Witness parent who has refused a blood transfusion for his or her child, the question posed and the response to it in the 2009 version of "Response from the Scripture" is quoted: "You're willing to let your child die because you refuse blood transfusions. I think that is terrible!"

"I can understand your point of view. I suppose you are imagining your own child in that situation. As parents we would do everything possible to safeguard our child's welfare, wouldn't we? So if folks like you and me were going to refuse some sort of medical treatment for our children, there would certainly have to be some compelling reason for it. Do you think that some parents might be influenced by what God's Word says here at Acts 15:28, 29? Do we have enough faith to do what God commands?"

Parental Authority over Minors

The following precepts are in the second edition of the Catechism of the Catholic Church:

2207—Authority, stability, and a life of relationships within the family constitute the foundation for freedom, security, and fraternity within society. The family is the community in which, from childhood, one can learn moral values, begin to honor God, and make good use of freedom. Family life is an initiation into society.

2209—The family must be helped and defended by appropriate social measures. Where families cannot fulfill these responsibilities, other social bodies have the duty of helping them and supporting the institution of the family. Following the principle of subsidiarity, larger communities should take care not to usurp the family's prerogatives or interfere in its life.

2211—The political community has a duty to honor the family, to assist it, and to ensure especially:

- The freedom to establish a family, have children, and bring them up in keeping with the family's own moral and religious convictions;

- The freedom to profess one's faith, to hand it on, and raise one's children in it, with the necessary means and institutions;

- The freedom to form associations with other families and so to have representation before civil authority.

2221—The fecundity of conjugal love cannot be reduced solely to the procreation of children, but must extend to their moral education and their spiritual formation. "The role of the parents in education is of such importance that it is almost impossible to provide an adequate substitute."

2222—Parents must regard their children as children of God and respect them as human persons. Showing themselves obedient to the will of the Father in Heaven, they educate their children to fulfill God's law.

2225—Through the grace of the sacrament of marriage, parents receive the responsibility and privilege of evangelizing their children. Parents should initiate their children at an early age into the mysteries of the faith of which they are the "first heralds" for their children. They should associate them from their tenderest years with the life of the Church. A wholesome family life can foster interior dispositions that are a genuine preparation for a living faith and remain a support for it throughout one's life.

2242—The citizen is obliged in conscience not to follow the directives of civil authorities when they are contrary to the demands of the moral order, to the fundamental rights of persons or the teachings of the Gospel. Refusing obedience to civil authorities, when their demands are contrary to those of an upright conscience, finds its justification in the distinction between serving God and serving the political community. "Render therefore to Caesar the things that are Caesar's, and to God the things that are God's." We must obey God rather than man.

Are these precepts not precisely what the Jehovah's Witnesses espouse? As a practicing Catholic, could I deny the same tenets to members of the Jehovah's Witness faith? My faith demands I accord to them the same definition of the role of parent as my religion's doctrines accord to me. These guiding doctrines shape my understanding of what is ethical and moral.

Right of Conscience, Morality, and Religious Freedom

Conscience is the judgment of the intellect and intuition that distinguishes right from wrong. Moral judgment is derived from values, norms, principals and rules. Most religions view conscience as being linked to the morality inherent in all human beings. The extent to which conscience informs moral judgment before an action is taken and whether such moral judgments should be based on reason is crucial to the concept of religious freedom.

Catholic theology sees conscience as the subjective norm of morality. The Catholic Church has only recently become aware of threats to its religious freedom and right of conscience—in the form of the contraception, abortifacient (abortion-inducing), and sterilization mandates that are part of the Patient Protection and Affordable Care Act imposed by the Obama Administration. To fulfill the mandates of this act, the United States Department of Health and Human Services developed a rule that would force virtually all private health insurance plans to provide coverage of these modalities—including plans offered by Catholic institutions and public programs funded by Catholic taxpayers. This rule violates the doctrines of the Catholic Church and the right of conscience of its members. Catholic teaching holds that, "Man has the right to act according to his conscience and in freedom so as personally to make moral decisions. He must not be forced to act contrary to his conscience. Nor must he be prevented from acting according to his conscience, especially in religious matters."

Do Jehovah's Witnesses deserve less? If you were to ask a Jehovah's Witness, "From where did conscience come?"—according to the 2009 version of "Response from the Scripture," he or she might respond:

"Belief in God is necessary to explain conscience in man. Why do we say that? Wherever and whenever men have lived, there has been an inborn sense of right and wrong, also sometimes called moral law or natural law, to guide their actions. However, some might argue that while one person using his conscience would call a certain practice entirely 'right,' another person would call it grossly 'wrong.' But inborn natural laws are those that consistently condemn the same basic wrongs in every society, such as murder and rape. From where did this universal natural law, moral law, or laws of conscience come? Do you know of any law that does not have a lawmaker? Furthermore, is it not reasonable that an outstandingly moral "person" must be the maker of a natural law that has worked for the obvious good and even preservation of all human society? That moral person is God."

Can the federal government enact a law that violates church teaching? The Jehovah's Witnesses began the battle over their constitutional rights, freedom of religion, and freedom of conscience in 1945. They have continued to hold the banner in the fight against government intrusions on conscience, particularly in the area of health care. They have not wavered in their longstanding commitment to act in accordance with their faith and moral values.

All religious institutions share equally in the same God-given, legally recognized right to not be forced to act in a manner contrary to their beliefs. At stake is religious freedom—the sacred right of any religious denomination to define its own teaching and ministry. Any attempt to reduce religious freedom to mere freedom of worship, without guarantees of respect for freedom of conscience, is to limit that most cherished of American freedoms. It is fitting that when the Bill of Rights was ratified, religious freedom had the distinction of being the first liberty described in that document.

James Madison, the father of the Constitution, described conscience as "the most sacred of all property." He wrote, "The Religion thereof of every man must be left to the conscience and conviction of every man; and it is the right of every man to exercise it as these may dictate." By authorizing a blood transfusion, the court fails to acknowledge the constitutionally protected rights of individual families and religious communities. The government has no business telling an American what to believe or how to act in regard to religious matters. By doing so, the government tramples on substantive constitutional rights. Invasion of the parent-child relationship and nonconsensual administration of medical treatment violate the fundamental right of parental authority. Should the values and preferences of the family or those of the doctor, hospital, or judge determine a child's medical care? Is the parent's choice to be respected only when the doctor agrees?

The conscience of the health care provider must also be respected. A clinician may not be comfortable with a patient's choices or with his or her ability to care for a Jehovah's Witness patient. If that is the case, the physician should consider referring the patient to another competent provider who is willing to assume care. We must respect the ethical and moral code of caregivers who profess difficulty in watching a child die from what they believe is a condition that can be successfully treated by blood transfusion.

What Do We Mean by Religious Liberty?

Religious liberty is the first liberty granted to us by God, and it is protected in the First Amendment to our Constitution:

"Congress shall make no law respecting an establishment of religion, or prohibiting the free exercise thereof; or abridging the freedom of speech, or of the press; or the right of the people peaceably to assemble and to petition the Government for a redress of grievances."

The phrase "shall make no law respecting an establishment of religion" started out as a prohibition on the power of Congress to either establish a national religion or to interfere with the established religions of the states. It has since been interpreted to forbid state establishment of religion, to forbid governmental preference (at any level) of one religion over another, and to forbid government funding of religion. The phrase "prohibiting the free exercise thereof" is generally used to protect citizens and institutions from government interference with the exercise of their religious beliefs. It sometimes is used to mandate the accommodation of religious practices when such practices conflict with federal, state or local laws.

Conclusion

It has been my experience in treating hundreds of Jehovah's Witnesses during my professional medical career that their firmly held conviction regarding the use of blood adds a degree of risk and may complicate their care. By the same token, they have sharpened my skills in seeking non-blood alternatives to conventional care. Honoring their religious beliefs despite criticism from my colleagues and unfriendly encounters with child protective services has become a badge of honor.

Witnesses manifest an unusual degree of appreciation and loyalty to a physician who respects and honors their disavowal of blood transfusions. In fact, their unusually high degree of compliance with my medical advice has been, I suspect, an effort to demonstrate acceptance of medical interventions to the extent their beliefs permit. Moreover, Jehovah's Witnesses have been the main impetus for the creation of bloodless surgery centers across the United States—centers where physicians practice alternatives to the use of blood transfusions, especially in the absence of an emergency situation or when the patient is not in critical condition. Unlike those who practice so-called faith healing, and who withhold medical treatment from themselves or their children, for Jehovah's Witnesses it is never no treatment but which treatment.

I have spent no sleepless nights during the more than three decades of my professional life as a result of honoring the requests of Witness parents to not transfuse their minor children, regardless of the nature or severity of their illnesses. To do otherwise would be the epitome of hypocrisy and a double standard for any medical professional who claims to respect the religious beliefs of patients. A consistent adherence to a code of ethics depends on systematic analyses of situations and focuses on the values and norms at stake. The ethically justified decisions and actions of physicians may violate the values and norms of Jehovah's Witness parents if the parents' firmly held religious tenets are violated when their child is transfused against their wishes.

In the United States, it is religion that is constitutionally protected from government and not the other way around. It is freedom of religion and not freedom from religion that we are privileged to enjoy in this country. Our nation was founded on the principles of equality and freedom. We have invested our resources and our lives to defend those principles, including the freedom to practice any religion of our choice.

I believe physicians who provide quality care without blood are not compromising their valued medical principles. Rather, these physicians show respect for the rights of patients to know all risks and benefits so patients can exercise their conscience in making informed choices regarding treatment, including making every attempt to preserve and protect the lives of their children from the moment of conception until natural death.

Some final thoughts: In the words of Cardinal Timothy Dolan, archbishop of New York, "The test of pluralism in a democracy is the protection afforded to minority views, especially of religious faith and practices."

In an op-ed published in the Wall Street Journal on February 12, 2013, George Weigel framed this issue succinctly: "...there can be neither true freedom nor true democracy without religious freedom in full. That means the right of both individuals of conscience and religious communities to live their lives according to their most deeply held convictions, and the right to bring those convictions into public life without civil penalty or cultural ostracism."

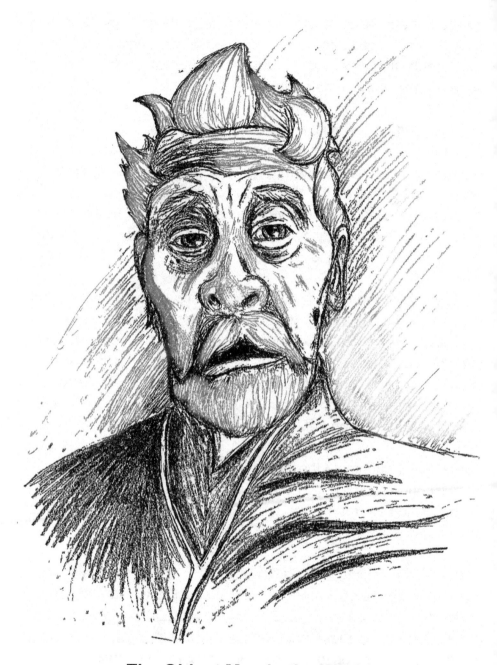

The Oldest Man in the World

In 1918, at the age of 15, Alexander and his classmates joined the Polish army to fight the Bolsheviks—returning to school in 1921. He married his childhood sweetheart. She left him a few years later for an artist. He retaliated by marrying her friend. In 1939, when the Nazis marched into Poland, he and his wife fled to Russian occupied Bialystok in northeast Poland. Refusing Soviet citizenship, they were sentenced to forced labor in the Abramkova gulag near the White Sea in northwest Russia. After two years of constant toil, small portions of often inedible food and subzero temperatures, they were sent to Samarkand in central Asia, today's Uzbekistan. When World War II ended, they made their way back to Poland only to discover that thirty members of their family perished in the Holocaust. His wife died, childless, in 1986.

Alexander Herbert Imich was born to an Ashkenazi Jewish family in Czestochowa, a city in southern Poland on February 4, 1903. Both of his parents lived into their 90s. Imich earned a PhD in zoology at the Jagiellonian University in Krakow, Poland, in 1929. Unable to further his academic career in zoology he turned to chemistry. Prior to immigrating to the United States in 1951, he was a senior chemist, plant manager and consultant in Poland, the USSR, Germany, and France. Alexander was fluent in all five languages of those countries. In the U.S., he worked in research labs and large industrial companies.

Since his teenage years, Alexander had a special interest in parapsychology, publishing more than 100 articles, reports and book reviews in Polish, Russian, East Indian, German, British and U.S. periodicals. In the early 1930s he began researching a Polish medium known as Matylda S. who was renowned for séances that reportedly called up the dead. Since retirement, he devoted himself to research on the occult and was the editor of a book entitled *Incredible Tales of the Paranormal: Documented Accounts of Poltergeist, Levitations, Phantoms and the Phenomena* published in 1995 at the age of 92. In this anthology, he also examined his special interest- psychokinetic phenomena from the Victorian era to modern experiments with psychic children in China. Psychokinesis is the ability to deform inanimate objects such as spoons and forks, mentally, or place objects into unopened bottles that would be impossible to insert through the opening at the top.

In 2007, after losing his life savings in a series of bad investments in the stock market, he was indigent and became dependent on community and voluntary social services for food. At age 104, the New York Times newspaper featured him as one of their neediest cases.

Imich was computer literate. He conducted voluminous research and correspondence on the Internet until the age of 110, when no longer able due to sight limitations imposed by age-related macular degeneration. Following a fall in his upper West Side Manhattan, New York, apartment, Alexander spent his 110th birthday in Roosevelt hospital, where he was rendered nearly deaf by losing both of his hearing aids.

Inspired by Eastern mystics, Imich ate sparingly, consuming mostly chicken and fish. He avoided alcohol and stopped smoking 50 years before he died. Athletic throughout his life, he described himself as a gymnast, a good runner and a good swimmer. At the age of 93, he prepaid a three year enrollment in a weekend school of the healing arts that emphasized personal development and relationships, self-mastery, self-awareness and learning to embody spiritual principals in one's life.

Alexander did not need full-time help until the last three months of his life. His condition deteriorated just two weeks before his death. He was medicated for agitation about four days before he died and died peacefully of natural causes on June 8, 2014, at the age of 111 years and 124 days. According to his medical directive, his body was turned over to Mount Sinai Medical Center for research. Imich's life was one of insatiable intellectual curiosity and ability to turn even great adversity into something positive. He believed the "neshama", the Hebrew word for soul or spirit, survives physical death.

Alexander Imich was the world's oldest man but not the oldest person. Sixty-six people, all women, are older, according to the organization, Gerontology Research. Misao Okawa of Osaka, Japan, is recognized as the world's oldest living person at 116 years of age. The rank of the world's oldest man now goes to Sakari Momoi of Fukushima, Japan. He was born just one day after Imich in 1903. Momoi is a survivor of the earthquake on March 11, 2011, that caused the meltdown of all three of Fukushima Prefecture's Daiichi nuclear power plants. The greatest fully-authenticated age to which any human has ever lived is 122 years, 164 days, reached by Jeanne Louise Calment of France.

Healthy Aging

"Healthy aging" and "successful aging" are usually defined as survival to 85 years and older and free from chronic diseases such as coronary heart disease, stroke, cancer and diabetes. These individuals continue to function well, both physically and cognitively, to age 94—nonagenarians. "Exceptionally healthy" older adults are those who take no medications; have well controlled chronic disease; no high blood pressure; and normal body weight who survive to age 95 and older. A study of almost 6,000 British civil service employees followed for 17 years found the strongest predictor of successful aging was socioeconomic position at mid-life. After adjusting for socioeconomics, not smoking, diet, exercise, moderate alcohol intake (in women) and work support (in men) predicted healthy aging. The environment, lifestyle and genetic factors contribute to successful aging as well as to longevity.

Longevity

Longevity is commonly thought of as typical or usual length of life. Genetic makeup, environmental exposures and lifestyle choices are major influences on one's longevity. From studies of identical and fraternal twins it has been determined genetics account for about 25 percent of the difference in longevity and environmental factors account for about 50 percent. The remainder is due to lifestyle, which can be modified and is likely to interact with genetics.

Life Expectancy

Life expectancy at birth among the U.S. population is defined as the average number of years remaining at a given age that a group of infants would live if the group was to experience, throughout life, the age-specific death rates present in their year of birth. For people born in 2012, life expectancy in the U.S. was at an all-time high of 76.4 years for men and 81.2 years for women, a difference of 4.8 years. To what can this improvement in life expectancy be attributed? According to a report issued in October 2014 by the National Center for Health Statistics of the Center for Disease Control and Prevention (CDC), the top ten causes of death in 2012 stayed the same as in 2011, but for 8 of the 10 the death rate fell significantly. Heart disease fell 1.8 percent; cancer fell 1.5 percent; chronic lower respiratory diseases fell 2.4 percent; stroke fell 2.6 percent; Alzheimer disease fell 3.6 percent; diabetes fell 1.9 percent; influenza and pneumonia fell 8.3 percent and kidney disease fell 2.2 percent. The suicide rate increased 2.4 percent and the rate remained the same for unintentional injury.

The average life expectancy for a person who was 65 years old in 2012 is 17.9 years for a man and 20.5 years for a woman—a difference of 2.6 years called the "female advantage." In that year, women were projected to reach age 85 and men age 83. It is not clear whether genetics plays a role in the life expectancy difference between the sexes but behavior probably does. Men take more risks and they participate in more dangerous outdoor activities. The older we get, the tighter the gap. If a man and a woman both reach 100, he is likely to live another month and she, four months.

Genetics

The genetic contribution to a healthy lifespan in those with exceptional longevity may be greater than in the general population. But is it possible those with exceptional longevity practice a healthy lifestyle or do longevity-associated genes protect them against the detrimental effects of an unhealthy lifestyle?

To answer these questions relevant to Alexander Imich, investigators at the Albert Einstein College of Medicine conducted a retrospective study of 477 Ashkenazi Jews ages 95 to 112 and their children, called the Longevity Genes Project. All those enrolled were community-dwelling and most were born in the U.S. or moved here before World War II. The genetic profile of Ashkenazi Jews traces their origins to just 250 to 420 ancestors in Central or Eastern Europe dating back 600 to 800 years ago. Preliminary findings in the study showed longevity is highly correlated to high HDL (high density lipoprotein)—good cholesterol—and low LDL (low density lipoprotein)—bad cholesterol levels. Certain mutations in cholesterol genes are associated with longevity and the prevention of cognitive decline and Alzheimer disease. CETP (cholesterol ester transfer protein), the product of a so-called longevity gene, was over-represented in the centenarians by nearly three-fold for 100 year olds compared to those in their seventh decade of life. The protein product of this gene is found in blood where it is involved in the transfer of cholesterol from HDL to other forms of cholesterol. How does it work? Perhaps by increasing the good cholesterol level and increasing the size of both high density and low density lipoproteins, CETP is protective against diabetes, high blood pressure and cardiovascular (heart and blood vessel) disease. Diabetes and Alzheimer disease was reduced by 80 percent in this group. Several genes have been found in the Ashkenazi associated with longevity, including mutations in a growth hormone gene resulting in lower growth hormone levels.

Surprisingly, 50 percent of those 100 years or older in the study were obese and 60 percent of the men and more than 40 percent of the women smoked cigarettes for more than 30 years. One woman had been smoking for 95 years. Exercise was moderate in this group. They did not interact with the environment in the way that we would want. A pattern of apparently healthy lifestyle was lacking. Those with exceptional longevity were not healthier in earlier life in terms of body mass index (BMI), smoking, physical activity or diet than the general U.S. population.

The Longevity Genes Project's observations support the notion that those with exceptional longevity may interact with the environment and lifestyle factors differently than others. It is generally acknowledged in the general population, environmental and lifestyle factors play a larger role in human lifespan than do genetic factors. For most people, interaction with the environment is important and a healthier lifestyle may enhance lifespan but it appears the presence of longevity genes in the Ashkenazi people with exceptional longevity cancels the presence of disease-associated genes. Yet, there was no difference in the presence of known disease-associated gene variants between the longevity group and the control group. It may be that the longevity genes help to interact with lifestyle more favorably than the rest of the population. If a particular gene prolongs life by protecting against cardiovascular disease, specifically by defending against the detrimental effects of smoking on the process of atherosclerosis, such a gene will be more common in people with exceptional longevity despite high smoking rates. This suggests people with exceptional longevity reach older ages despite lifestyle choices similar to those of the general population, supporting the notion that genetic factors related to exceptional longevity may also protect against the detrimental effects of poor lifestyle choices. Naturally, this analysis may be peculiar to Ashkenazi Jews and not reflective of the population in general.

In the New England Centenarian study, the largest study of centenarians in the world, researchers at Boston University looked at a representative cross-section of the Caucasian population and identified genes associated with living longer in 1,500 centenarians compared to 1,267 people who were not yet 100. As much as possible, they matched the genetic backgrounds of the centenarians to the comparison group (controls) and were able to predict, using genetics alone, many of those who would be a centenarian. The scientists identified 150 DNA sequence variations called single nucleotide polymorphisms (SNPs) among those 100 years old and above that may have contributed to their healthy aging. See the section on genetics in the chapter entitled Wombmates for a detailed explanation of this phenomenon. Fifteen percent had longevity associated genes. In theory, 15 percent of the American population is predisposed to live to be 100. They were able to predict with 77 percent accuracy who would live to be 100 or higher, based on genetics alone. That means there are 23 percent of centenarians who do not have the right genetic makeup. Apparently, environmental and lifestyle factors are still relevant. Surprisingly, they found little difference between the centenarians and the controls in terms of the number of genetic variants associated with diseases of aging, cardiovascular disease, stroke and Alzheimer disease.

Perhaps what makes centenarians live longer is not a lack of predisposition to such illnesses but the enrichment of genetic variants associated with longevity. The longevity-associated genes may be cancelling out the negative effects of the genes linked to disease. Current gene profiling does not take into account those longevity genes that may override the genes that are linked to disease. Recent studies attempting to clarify the genetic basis of longevity confirm that only variants of two genes—apolipoprotein E (APOE) and forkhead box 03A (FOXO3A)—are consistently associated with longevity. APOE is a major carrier of cholesterol and supports fat transport and injury repair in the brain. FOX03A is involved with insulin sensitivity, perhaps preventing diabetes.

It is also possible epigenetic factors may contribute to exceptional longevity. Life is much more complicated than the sequences of our DNA. Stresses placed on people at different times of their lives influence gene expression. Over the course of their lives, individuals methylate their DNA at different rates—see the section on epigenetics in the chapter, Wombmates, for a detailed explanation of this phenomenon.

Environment

Environmental quality is a very important factor affecting sickness and health. Air and water pollution, depletion of natural resources and soil deterioration are all capable of increasing the death rate, thereby reducing longevity. Environmental factors are believed to represent half the contributions to longevity.

Lifestyle

Lifestyle choices, particularly diet, exercise and smoking habits, play an undisputed role in determining not only how long one will live but how well one will age. A study of the regions of the world where people commonly live active lives past 100 years of age, speculated that longevity is related to a healthy social and family life, not smoking, eating a plant-based diet, frequent consumption of legumes and nuts, and engaging in regular physical activities. This combination accounted for a difference of up to 10 years in life expectancy. Even modest amounts of physical exercise can increase lifespan by as much as 4.5 years. The five longevity virtues are regular exercise; not smoking, moderate alcohol consumption; maintaining a low body mass index and eating a predominantly plant-based diet. If one practices four or five of those virtues compared with those who practice none, the reduction in cardiovascular disease is 67 percent; diabetes 73 percent; cancer 20-25 percent; dementia 65 percent; and all-cause deaths 32 percent.

According to the Dietary Guidelines for Americans, moderate alcohol consumption is defined as having one drink per day for women and up to two drinks per day for men. A standard drink is equal to 14 grams (0.6 ounces) of pure alcohol. This amount is found in 12 ounces of beer with 5 percent alcohol content; 8 ounces of malt liquor with 7 percent alcohol content; 5 ounces of wine with 12 percent alcohol content; 1.5 ounces or a shot of 80-proof (40 percent alcohol content) distilled spirits or liquor such as gin, rum, vodka or whiskey. It is the amount of alcohol consumed, not the type of alcoholic drink.

In several interviews, Alexander Imich suggested that not having children may have contributed to his longevity. The Longevity Genes Project observed that both male and female Ashkenazi Jewish centenarians born around the turn of the century, who reached reproductive age in the 1920s, had a smaller number of children than a contemporaneous population with usual survival. They also tended to reproduce later in life. It is unclear whether these observations can be generalized to other ethnicities since the responsible mechanism may be unrecognized genetic factors peculiar to Ashkenazi Jews. When asked to what he attributed his longevity, Alexander responded "To the fact that I haven't died."

Centenarians

Only one in 10,000 lives to be 100 years of age—a centenarian. The United States currently has the greatest number of known centenarians of any nation with 53,364 according to the 2010 Census or 17.3 per 100,000 people, an increase of 65.8 percent since 1980. Of these, 82.8 percent were female. In some countries, the ratio of female to males who live to be 100 or more is quite variable. It ranges from 2 to 1 in Sardinia to 7 to 1 in northern Italy, suggesting a gene-environment interaction. By 2050, the number of centenarians is expected to hit 600,000. In that year, the average lifespan will be in the mid-80s, up from 77.85 in 2006. In the year

2100, the US Census Bureau predicts there will be 5.3 million people over 100 years of age.

A supercentenarian is a person who has lived to the age of 110 or more, achieved by about one in 1,000 centenarians. Even rarer is a person who has lived to the age of 115. There are only 34 people in recorded history who have indisputably reached this age. All of those still living are females.

The highest concentration of centenarians in the world is found in Okinawa, Japan. Their longevity is attributed to a calorie restricted diet which is optimally nutritious. Not surprising, there is exceptional longevity in the parents, siblings and offspring of their centenarians suggesting a genetic contribution to their longevity. The population of Okinawa is very homogeneous in its ethnic and racial composition compared to the United States and provides a better platform upon which to study the influence of environmental and behavioral factors. In both the U.S. and Okinawa environmental and lifestyle influence a person's likelihood of living to their mid-80s but in the extremes of old age, genetics play more of a role.

As a group, 100 year olds are not 80 year olds who have tacked on 20 years of physical and mental decline. Instead, centenarians typically do not suffer chronic illnesses associated with age until shortly before dying or escape them altogether. Of those who make it to 100, more than 90 percent are physically and mentally healthy at the age of 93 and about half live on their own or with family. They have many friends, strong ties to relatives and higher self-esteem. Those who have been through traumatic life events are more likely to reach centenarian status. Perhaps the philosopher, Friedrich Nietzsche, was right when he said, "What doesn't kill you make you stronger."

Longevity Predictions in Healthcare

Longevity predictions are important in many aspects of medical care, especially to health insurers and to some basic premises in the Affordable Care Act upon which premiums are based. Centenarians tend to stay healthy and die quickly. According to current CDC data, medical costs in the final two years of life were $24,000 for those who died when they were 60 to 70 years of age and one-third as much—$8,000—for those who died when they were older than 100. Surely, these costs go up proportionately each year.

Physicians are concerned about a national healthcare policy in which treatment is restricted just based on age. Relying on age alone, without additional factors such as frailty, quality of life and concurrent diseases, is something we must avoid. Besides, the organs of the same person age at different rates.

Limited survival will impact the benefits of initiating medications or performing screening tests and procedures. Decision-making regarding the appropriateness of specific interventions is impacted.

Should a 75 year old be given medication to prevent osteoporosis? That decision requires recognition of the likely survival time of the individual and how long it will take for the medication to have an effect.

People older than 80 years comprise an increasing segment of the population with elevated cholesterol levels and risk of cardiovascular disease. Because there is substantial biologic and functional variation among older patients, the decision for the use of statin medications differs in older patients relative to younger ones. A review of the medical literature in September 2014 concluded there are no randomized clinical trials of statins or any medications for elevated cholesterol that included persons older than 80 years at the start of the trial. Findings in 75 to 80 year olds support statin treatment for prevention of atherosclerotic (marked by cholesterol plaques) cardiovascular disease (ASCVD) and probably in diabetics without ASCVD. Harm from statin drugs are is not increased in older people so their use in prevention is possible but should be started before age 80. Because people older than 80 are functionally and biologically different, have varying life expectancy, may have frailty or concurrent illnesses and may take multiple medications, the decision to treat with statins must be individualized but is not supported by high quality evidence.

An 85 year old man has pain attributable to a hernia in his groin. It could become strangulated—losing the blood supply to that portion of his intestine caught in the hernia—and develop gangrene. The problem is not likely to go away in the next 4.7 years of his estimated life expectancy. This obviously warrants the decision to perform the surgical repair.

The reason physicians study the aging process is not to make people live longer but for them to have a healthier lifespan. For the one in 10,000 who is ordained to live to a triple digit age, we should not be hesitant about proceeding with indicated medical treatment or surgical procedures after the age of 75.

A final thought: If only we could predict exceptional longevity as well as we know how to reduce the disease risks that shorten longevity.

About the Author

Dr. Augustine L. Perrotta is a Clinical Professor of Medicine-Emeritus at Michigan State University College of Osteopathic Medicine, Clinical Professor of Exercise Science at Oakland University and Master Fellow of the American College of Osteopathic Internists. He is board certified in internal medicine, hematology, medical oncology, clinical and applied thrombosis, hemostasis and vascular medicine and is certified in sedation and analgesia. Dr. Perrotta is the author or co-author of 50 articles and abstracts in the medical literature. He is president of the Birmingham/Bloomfield Affiliate of Right to Life of Michigan, member of the John Paul II Bioethics Commission and chairman of the Visitation-Health Committee of the Senior Men's Club of Birmingham.

For more information,
http://stephaniecampbellreleases.weebly.com/
CaseClosedBook@hotmail.com

Find more books from
Keith Publications, LLC
At

www.keithpublications.com

9 781628 820935